HUNGRY

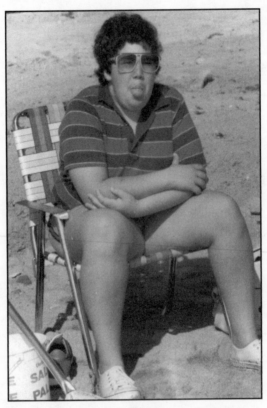

Allen Zadoff at the beach, age fifteen

HUNGRY

Lessons Learned
ON THE
Journey
FROM
Fat to Thin

ALLEN ZADOFF

Da Capo

LIFE
LONG
A Member of the Perseus Books Group

Copyright © 2007 by Allen Zadoff

Designed by Brent Wilcox
Set in 11.5 point Kepler MM by the Perseus Books Group

Library of Congress Cataloging-in-Publication Data
Zadoff, Allen.
   Hungry : lessons learned on the journey from fat to thin / Allen Zadoff.—1st Da Capo Press ed.
     p. cm.
  ISBN-13: 978-0-7382-1105-3 (alk. paper)
  ISBN-10: 0-7382-1105-2 (alk. paper)
   1. Zadoff, Allen—Mental health. 2. Compulsive eaters—United States—Biography. 3. Overweight men—United States—Biography. I. Title.
RC552.C65Z33 2007
362.196'85260092—dc22
[B]

2007007517

Published by Da Capo Press
A Member of the Perseus Books Group
www.dacapopress.com

Note: Some of the names and identifying details of people associated with events described in this book have been changed. Any similarity to actual persons is coincidental.

CONTENTS

CONTENTS

CONTENTS

PART 4
What I Know Now   127

CONTENTS

INTRODUCTION

From the time I was a young boy, I loved to eat. It began at six years old when I locked myself in my room with a box of Devil Dogs. While other kids were playing kick-the-can and dodge-ball in the dead end at the base of our neighborhood hill, I was watching cartoons in my bedroom and chewing. I don't know why Devil Dogs were so special to me. I only know that the combination of white cream and spongy chocolate cake was indeed devilish. One bite of the dog, and I was transported. It was as if the dog had bitten me rather than the reverse. I lost entire afternoons in the clutch of its jaws, obsessed by the crinkling of plastic packaging, the sucking of cream, the licking of cake, the scraping of wet chocolate from the roof of my mouth. I thought eating Devil Dogs was a wonderful thing, marred only by the necessity of hiding them from my mother, who even then was concerned about my weight.

Once I had mastered the dogs, I quickly moved on to other foods, such as Reese's Peanut Butter Cups, Drakes Coffee

Cakes, and Lenders Bagels. I became something like a magician with my mouth. I could eat the peanut butter from the center of the cup without touching the chocolate, scrape the cinnamon topping from the coffee cake while saving the cake for later, and eat bagel after bagel without getting full. Eventually, my mouth could make large pizzas disappear without anyone knowing how I did it.

Of course, all this eating had an unintended effect: I got fat. Really fat.

By my midtwenties, I had topped out somewhere around 360 pounds, not quite the size of a Macy's float, but well on my way.

How does someone get to be 360 pounds?

Um . . . one pound at a time.

I'm only half joking. Nobody starts out thinking they're going to be fat. When I was a pudgy child, I was sure I would never get above 200 pounds, despite the fact that the buttons on my Cub Scout uniform kept drifting suspiciously apart. When I was a teen, I was convinced I would never weigh 250, at least until I stepped on a scale at sixteen years old and saw the arm balance out at 272. I immediately signed up for Weight Watchers with my dad's help. I was certain I would lose weight and be thin forever.

I did lose weight, for about an hour. Then I started eating Devil Dogs, Doritos, and other foods again. I couldn't help it. They were too delicious to give up forever. And truth be told, I was kind of lonely without them.

All the time I was eating, I was desperate to get thin. At first I thought thin would just happen to me without my doing anything. Like puberty. One day you're walking down the street, and POW! Hormones. I figured getting thin would happen the same way. I'd wake up one morning, and Thin would be waiting for me in the mirror.

"Hello, Thin, I've been expecting you for quite a while."

"Sorry, Allen, I got held up at Brad Pitt's house. But I'm here now. Are you ready to start your modeling career?"

"Sure!"

But Thin was not waiting for me. Something else was.

I passed 300 pounds at a sprint during college. I was less and less certain that I would ever be skinny. It was hard to claim I was still suffering from baby fat at twenty-two years old. I began to resign myself to life as a fat man. Not just any fat man, but a really fat one. My father also struggled with his weight, but his weight never seemed to rise above a certain moderately uncomfortable level. My own fat was different. It had ambition. It was not going to be limited by size 42 pants or XL shirts. It wanted more. And so it climbed to 325, then 350. My waistline swelled to size 54, my shirts to 4XL. Four hundred pounds was a virtual certainty.

And then, suddenly, it all changed.

The best way I can describe it is to say that food stopped working.

Over the years, eating had always provided me a great sense of relief, comfort, and release. Of course, I hated myself after eating, but the lead-up to the first bite was as near as I came to heaven on earth. There was nothing better than driving home with a bag of hot food in the seat beside me. Having Chinese leftovers in my refrigerator made me feel safe, like a food 401k.

But at age twenty-eight, for reasons I would understand only much later, the pleasure went away. The more I ate, the worse I felt. The taste hadn't changed, but the joy was gone. I was now overeating not for pleasure but because I couldn't stop myself. When I looked back over my life, I saw that it had been that way for a long time. From the beginning, I had been seeking skinny and finding fat. If there was any other way to live, I didn't know what it was.

This crisis, so frightening at the time, turned out to be the greatest opportunity of my life. I knew it was time to change, but I didn't know how to begin.

I knew what not to do. I didn't go on a diet, and I didn't get on a scale. I didn't give my credit card to a skinny woman in a lab coat. I didn't join a gym and try to exercise the calories away. I'd done all those things before, over and over, and they'd never worked as more than a temporary solution.

Instead, I sought help not to control my weight but to deal with the emotional turmoil that was lurking just beneath the food. It wasn't normal to spend Saturday night alone making love to a three-cheese pizza. As far as I knew, normal people didn't hide food in their pockets and up their sleeves so other people wouldn't see them eating. It didn't seem right that I was twenty-eight, without a girlfriend, without a career, with nothing like true friendships. I'd always attacked my weight problem head-on, but now I started to explore the world behind the food.

Over the course of a year, more than 100 pounds fell from my body, and my thin life, the one I'd been waiting nearly thirty years for, finally began. It was nothing like I expected. For starters, Calvin Klein did not call with a modeling offer. The gifts of the thin life, which I'd always assumed included a beautiful wife, gorgeous house, and handsome Labrador retriever, did not materialize. My life was not suddenly perfect. It was a lot more interesting than that. It turned out that losing weight was only the first step in a much larger and more amazing journey.

Going from fat to thin was like opening a door to another world. I didn't understand the thin life until I was already living it, and I couldn't clearly see my fat life until I'd passed beyond it and could look back.

All the years I was fat, I thought it was my fault, a combination of lack of willpower, weak character, and love of food. No doctor, therapist, or nutritionist—no matter how sincere— was able to give me the information I needed to be able to change. Ironically, it wasn't until I was already thin that I learned what I'd needed to know.

This book is what I wish I'd known all those years.

I spent twenty-eight years building up a set of beliefs about myself, my weight, and food, and I've worked for twelve years to tear it down. Losing 150 pounds was only the beginning.

Here is a little of what I learned along the way.

PART ONE

What I Believed on the Way Up the Scale

"When you wake up in the morning, Pooh," said Piglet at last, *"what's the first thing you say to yourself?"*

"What's for breakfast?" said Pooh. "What do you say, Piglet?"

"I say, I wonder what's going to happen exciting today?" said Piglet.

Pooh nodded thoughtfully.

"It's the same thing," he said.

Winnie-the-Pooh by A. A. Milne

If I Wasn't Fat,
I'd Be Happy

At 360 POUNDS, I clung to the myth of thin like a drowning man grasping a life preserver. It went something like this:

If I was thin, I'd be happy.

What else could I believe? Life at an enormous weight was a never-ending cycle of rejection, shame, and mortification, punctuated by the all-too-brief ecstasy of eating huge and delicious combinations of sugar, salt, and grease. With pain as my constant companion, I had to believe there was something on the other side, something wonderful, something that would make all the pain and frustration of living fat worthwhile.

This something was the Thin Life. It was my version of heaven.

Never having been thin, you might wonder how I knew so much about thin people and their happiness.

I had read the J.Crew catalog.

From time to time, the J.Crew catalog would appear in my mailbox in New York. (It was addressed to the previous resident. I never actually went into a J.Crew store until years later when I had slimmed down to a near-normal weight.) I combed the pages of the catalog, studying scenes of city, sand, and sea. Here were the thin men I wanted to be, the thin women I wanted to date, the thin pants I wanted to fit into. These thin people were laughing and smiling and holding hands as they walked on the beach. They slung leather satchels over their shoulders and strolled arm in arm as they browsed at the local farmers market. They smiled at each other across a café table as they sipped cappuccino and talked thin-people talk.

I wasn't completely naïve. I knew that pictures in a catalog weren't the same thing as real life. But when I looked around the so-called real world, I saw more or less the same thing that was in the magazine.

From the time I was a young boy, thin people always looked happy to me. Thin kids loved gym and recess, while I resented it. Thin kids ate delicious snacks in the cafeteria where everyone could see them. They didn't have to hide or feel ashamed like I did. Thin families laughed and played together, while my overweight family argued and worried.

During high school, thin people played sports, went to dances, and always had somewhere to be on Friday night. During college, thin people went out drinking and experimented with sex.

By the time I made it to Manhattan in my midtwenties, thin people had added jobs, cars, and sophisticated love affairs to their repertoire. I'd added cable television and Chinese food delivered to my tiny Manhattan apartment.

The Thin Life was all around me—on the streets, on television, in the pages of magazines—and it looked delicious.

If I wasn't fat, I would be living the Thin Life.

Then I would be happy, just like them.

I Have to Find
the Perfect Diet

I WENT ON PLENTY of diets in my life: Weight Watchers, Scarsdale, Slim Fast, Diet Center, Jenny Craig, Medifast. They all worked for a while, but then my willpower failed me. At least I assumed it was my willpower. Why else would I stop doing what was obviously helping me lose weight?

I went to various doctors in search of answers. They handed me faded photocopies of diet plans that told me to take one piece of bread off my sandwich and never eat after 8 PM. Then they'd pat me on the shoulder and say, "If you want to lose weight badly enough, you will. You can do anything you set your mind to." So I set my mind. But every time I modified my eating with a diet, life became unbearable. When I inevitably went back to eating the old way, there were only two things I could assume: either I wasn't strong enough to do the diet or the diet itself was faulty.

In my mind, the perfect diet would allow for rapid weight loss while somehow overcoming the hopeless lack of willpower that plagued me every time I tried to change my eating habits.

Each new diet promised that it would solve this riddle. "On our plan, you'll never be hungry!" the ads shouted. But I was always hungry. It didn't matter how much food the diet allowed or how many delicious snacks were built into the framework. Anything less than an all-out food binge was unsatisfying to me.

As the professionals got a little more savvy over the years, I began to hear some chatter about diets not being the answer. The new thinking told me I had to permanently change my relationship with food. It made sense to me, so I went to the doctor again.

We sat in his office, a set of weight-loss pamphlets spread across the mahogany desk in front of me.

"How do I do it?" I asked him. "How do I permanently change my relationship with food?"

"Eat less and exercise more," he told me.

My hopes fell. That was like telling a drowning man that in order to stop drowning, he has to think less about water.

"You can't think of it like a diet," he said. "It's forever."

"Forever?" I said.

"Absolutely." He passed me a pamphlet.

I walked from his office, tears forming in my eyes. I couldn't eat less forever. Chances were I couldn't even eat less for lunch that day.

If I Learn Why I Eat,
I'll Be Able to Stop

I WAS FIFTEEN YEARS old at a theater camp run by members of an off-Broadway theater troupe, the Circle Repertory Company. It was the dream of a lifetime, training with professionals, getting my first taste of the big-time theater world in New York City. In the middle of the summer, my acting teacher called me in for an evaluation.

"You're a fabulous actor," she said, "but you're heavy, and I have to be honest with you: at your current weight, you'll never be cast as a leading man. You're doomed to be a character actor your entire life."

Like most young actors, I was planning to be Robert Redford, so the news did not sit well with me.

"There's something else," she said. "You won't be able to get work until you're thirty-five years old. That's the age when character actors start to get roles."

This was getting worse and worse. First she'd told me I was fat, then she'd said I'd never be a star, and now I was evidently going to have to wait twenty years to get a job.

"What can I do?" I said, panic rising in my voice.

"There's only one possibility," she said. "You have to find out why you're eating so much. If you find out why you're eating, you'll be able to stop."

Her words hit me like a news flash. There was a reason I ate too much? The idea had never occurred to me. It was true that I ate more than the other kids, but I thought it was because . . .

Well, I'd never really thought about it. I was busy focusing on how fat I was. Being a fat kid, you do a lot of ducking and dodging, protecting yourself from the cruelty of kids at recess, in gym class, at the beach. There's not a lot of time for self-reflection.

My teacher's idea was new and exciting. I ate too much, and there was a reason behind it. My teacher had to be right. So I spent the next thirteen years trying to figure out the reason.

I started that very summer. I wasn't exactly self-aware at fifteen—more like self-conscious. But I did my best to pay attention to my overeating and to guess why I did it. What did I find out?

I ate because kids made fun of me. I felt ashamed, and I had a snack to feel better. When my parents pissed me off, I went to my room and had some Doritos. I also ate because girls liked the jocks better than they liked me. Then again, my first girlfriend, Julia, had kissed me on the lips that summer, and I was so excited, I ate extra dessert that night, stuffing myself with ice cream while I played the kiss over and over again in my mind.

Sometimes I ate simply because food was delicious. Who in their right mind would turn down a double-fudge brownie or a freshly baked chocolate chip cookie? Other times I ate for social reasons. If normal kids had an ice cream party, I wanted to join the party, too, preferably with a can of whipped cream in my hand. When the thin actors hopped out of bed to grab a late-night snack, I hopped, too. Why not?

As best I could tell, I overate pretty much anytime I could get away with it.

For the next ten years, the circumstances changed, but the reasons for my overeating did not. I ate when I got an A on a test and when I didn't, when a girl talked to me in a bar or when she didn't, when college was over and I was sad and when graduate school started and I was happy. I ate when I became a director and my productions earned me a lot of attention. I ate when a production was poorly reviewed and I got no attention.

Through it all, I clung to my teacher's idea that knowing why I overate would set me free.

Beware of Exploding Donuts

LATER ON, a well-meaning dietitian added another in-gredient to the mix. She asked me to look for situations that caused me to overeat, such as being stressed, meeting new people, or getting too busy at work. If I could identify these sit-uations, she said, I could learn to recognize them as they were happening, then defuse them before they caused me to overeat and damage myself. The process was something like pulling a burning fuse out of a stick of dynamite. First you have to know how dynamite works, then you have to notice when the fuse is lit, and then you have to yank hard before it blows up in your face.

I did what she told me to do. I kept a diary of situations that made me want to overeat for a week, shared it with her, then set about recognizing and yanking fuses in pursuit of my new TNT-free lifestyle.

It was a great idea, and it worked for a while, but eventually the need to overeat became more powerful than the desire to pull the fuse. I'd notice the kind of situation she described—arguing with my mother on the phone, for instance—but instead of drinking a glass of water, taking a walk, or calling a friend like the dietitian suggested, I just went to the refrigerator and ate the second shelf. Boom.

Eventually, I stopped paying attention altogether. My entire life seemed to make me want to eat, and knowing that fact didn't help me at all. There was nothing I could do but bounce from situation to situation, overeat, then hate myself for my weakness. With fried chicken and bagels exploding all around me, I moved on to the next diet idea.

Tupperware Will Save Me

THE COUNSELORS AT another commercial diet plan explained how bad habits were conspiring to unhinge my potentially healthy eating. I had to plan better, they said, and stop making food choices in the moment. For example, they said I could bake six chicken breasts at the beginning of the week, put them in individual bags in the freezer, then defrost one bag a night with some steamed vegetables. Voilà! I'd have an instant, easily prepared meal instead of another trip to the McDonald's drive-through.

I understood the concept, and I planned. I filled my freezer. I carried half-ounce bags of cashews with me. I put carrot sticks in Tupperware containers and slipped them into my backpack. I scheduled my meals at proper intervals. I measured portions.

I cheated. I got fatter.

No surprise. Imagine me at 250 pounds, pulling out six measly cashews and a carrot stick for a midafternoon snack. It was enough to make a fat man cry.

All these diet plans were trying to help me, and they all gave me decent information about why I overate.

They said I ate because of my feelings. Because of things that happened in my past. Because of food triggers. Because of bad habits and poor planning.

All good ideas. All true to some extent. All useless to me.

I hopscotched from idea to idea, stubbornly holding to the belief that the real secret of why I ate lay just around the next corner and, when I came across it, I would recognize it and use it to be able to stop.

Maybe I'm Big-Boned

"MAYBE I'M FAT because I'm big-boned," I thought.

I'd heard my mother say as much when I was younger. I didn't know what *big-boned* meant exactly, but I guessed that it had to do with genetics. If I was born with bigger bones, then my body needed more weight in order to sustain them. My size, therefore, was the natural result of being born into a fat family. I was genetically predisposed to be larger than my peers.

I compared myself to an elephant. "Is an elephant fat," I asked myself, "or does it just look like an elephant is supposed to look?" The way I saw it, everyone in the world was at the mercy of the genetic lottery. If you won the lottery, you were born a cheetah. If you lost, you were an elephant.

I was an elephant. I was big-boned. End of story.

Maybe I Have a
Slow Metabolism

WHAT A RELIEF to find out I had a slow metabolism.

Nobody had told me that, but I was looking forward to the day when the medical establishment would perform a test and find out it was true. The doctor would call me into his office with a smile on his face.

"Allen," he'd say, "we've found the problem. It's glandular."

"Which gland?" I'd say.

"It doesn't matter. What matters is that being fat is not your fault."

At last, I'd find out what I'd secretly believed: All the years of struggling had been for naught. My body had a chemical imbalance, and it had caused my metabolism to slow down.

"Now the good news," the doctor would say. "We've got a pill to fix you."

He would write me a prescription, and that would be that. I could take the pill every day, and without dieting, feeling hungry, or struggling, the weight would fall from my body, and I would be thin. Once and for all.

Maybe I Don't Have
Enough Willpower

I WAS A REASONABLY smart guy. I got all As in high school, and I had a graduate degree from Harvard. I could read and understand nearly anything put in front of me. I could analyze problems and find solutions. When people spoke to me, I listened and understood.

So why was it that when doctors gave me diets, I could read them but I couldn't stay on them? I understood very well that 3,500 calories equals one pound, and if I reduced my caloric intake by 500 calories a day, I would lose one pound per week.

I read the Weight Watchers pamphlets, but I couldn't do what they told me to do. I knew it was imperative to stay on their diet, any diet, but I inevitably dropped out and started overeating again.

I wasn't stupid, so there had to be another reason.

I was weak.

What else could it be? I was lazy and weak. You had to be strong to stay on a diet. You had to be tough. Eventually, you'd want cookies when you were supposed to want carrots. That was inevitable. The real question was what you would do when that happened. When things got difficult and you wanted to eat, would you be tough and bite the carrot or weak and bite the cookie?

When it came to my personal struggle of cookies versus carrots, carrots might win the occasional battle, but cookies always won the war.

Maybe I'm Hungry

I FELT HUNGRY almost all the time.

I was hungry for salty things, then sweet things, rich things, then greasy things. Sometimes I was hungry for cold, other times hot. To start, I wanted crunchy; later, I wanted creamy.

The only time I wasn't hungry was when I was full. More than full. Stuffed.

This was how I did it: The moment I felt hungry, I ate until I was stuffed. The moment I was less than stuffed, I felt hungry again. Then I repeated the process.

I naturally assumed I was hungrier than other people. Other people weren't fat. Other people could stop before finishing the package of cookies, potato chips, or ice cream sandwiches. Other people weren't tortured by food thoughts, so they must not be hungry in the same way as me.

If I wasn't so hungry, I would be thin. That's what I believed.

Real Men Eat Nachos

WHEN I WAS growing up, men didn't have issues with food. If a man ate too much and gained a little weight, he was supposed to do some exercise until it melted off or morphed into muscle. He certainly wasn't supposed to worry about it, feel self-conscious, or discuss it with anyone.

Men were expected to eat a lot. They even named a frozen dinner after us. It was called Hungry Man, and it was the biggest frozen dinner on the market. A big, healthy man had a big appetite. He was hungry, and there was no shame in that. Quite the opposite. There was pride.

The era of the eating disorder was just coming into vogue when I was in high school. The *After-School Specials* of the time featured stories of anorexic and bulimic teenage girls who were hell-bent on harming themselves with food and exercise. If you had asked me my definition of an eating disorder at the time, I would have said it was something a cute sixteen-year-old girl did in her closet with food.

My own food and weight problems, obvious even in high school when I weighed 272 pounds, did not rise to the level of "disorder" in my mind. My diagnosis? I was simply what my teen peers called a "fat shit."

As time went on and I got fatter, it never occurred to me that something might be seriously wrong with me. I just could not believe that I, as a man, might have a problem with food. I had a problem with weight. I had a problem with willpower. But it wasn't food, and it certainly wasn't an eating disorder. Men didn't have eating disorders; they had Superbowl parties. They ordered hot wings and nachos and sat around with other men stuffing their faces and shouting at the TV screen.

Men knew how to handle their weight, and as far as I was concerned, I should be able to handle mine.

Even Santa Claus Was Jolly

AT 360 POUNDS, everyone seemed happier than me. That might have been because I was miserable.

I'd known for a long time that thin people were happy. They laughed, ate together, held hands, went to the gym. That was no great surprise.

I was a lot more upset by the fact that when I looked at fat people, they too seemed happy. They smiled when they waddled down the street. They said hello to people in stores. They ordered in restaurants and bought things in the deli while smiling and talking to the cashier. It's true that they didn't have cute girlfriends and boyfriends like the thin people, but it didn't seem to faze them. They still went out into the world and interacted with the inhabitants of planet earth.

I did not. I hid inside the house, ate secretly, thought secret thoughts.

Fat people were supposed to be my comrades in arms, but they didn't seem like me at all. I'd rather be caught dead than be seen walking down the street eating an ice cream cone, yet when summer rolled around, fat people hit the streets eating ice cream like it was no big deal. At Christmastime, fat people put on red suits and laughed while giving out gifts at the mall.

I looked to other fat people for recognition that I wasn't alone. Instead, I found yet another reason to feel isolated, depressed, and confused.

If You Could Only
See the Real Me . . .

As a fat person, I blamed all my failings on my weight. When I was unhappy or lonely or unsuccessful, it was because I was fat. When a pretty girl failed to be interested in me, it wasn't me she was rejecting, but the weight. When I didn't get a job, it was because the job discriminated against fat people. Whatever problems I had and whatever rejections I received could be traced back to my weight.

As I saw it, my fat was like an ugly shell that surrounded me. It was not the real me. The real me was hidden inside, and he was handsome, sexy, and amazing. He had a full social calendar and was scheduled to appear in *GQ* sometime soon.

Still, when I looked in the mirror, my fat was staring back at me. Trying to make the best of a bad situation, I decided to think of my fat as a sophisticated screening device. If you rejected me because I was fat, it spoke poorly of you. If you weren't capable of seeing through the ugly exterior to the inner *GQ* model, then you were a superficial idiot who didn't deserve my time or attention.

That's the story I told myself. The problem was that deep inside, I knew I was kidding myself.

You Have to Dodge the Delivery Guy

CHINESE DELIVERY WAS on the way. I counted out my money and a tip before the delivery guy got there, so I'd have to open the door for only the briefest of moments. I turned up the TV so he might think there was more than one person in the apartment. I put on sweatpants so I'd be presentable.

I realized I was staging things so they'd look good for a delivery guy I didn't know. It was crazy, but I couldn't help myself. I needed to look normal for the fifteen-second interaction when I got my stash. I needed to look normal even though I was more than 300 pounds, alone on a Friday night, ordering enough food for three people.

The buzzer rang, and I rushed to the door. The deal went down without a hitch. I briefly thought the delivery guy was watching me, judging me, wondering what the hell I was doing eating so much food.

The truth is, I was the only one thinking that. He was just worried about his tip.

Elated, I spread my stash out on the table in front of the television. Sesame noodles, dumplings, chicken and broccoli, fried rice, almond cookies. I dug in, eating at a furious pace. I imagined my hands were a blur, like Superman in the movie when he flies around the world to try to save Lois Lane. I was trying to save myself, and eating was the only way I knew how to do it. The food, which had seemed so abundant when I unpacked it, disappeared at a heartbreaking pace.

Totally stuffed, I settled down on the couch and unbuckled my pants. I was back in my comfort zone: sofa, kitchen, bathroom—the overeater's Bermuda Triangle.

Hide and Sneak

I WAS REASONABLY CERTAIN that I was the only one in the world who ate in such an ugly, secretive manner. The fat clients at the commercial diet centers talked about craving and sneaking food, things that were certainly familiar to me, but their behavior sounded pretty mild compared to my average Friday night.

By my midtwenties, I was buying increasingly large amounts of food and eating it while hiding in my apartment. I was polishing off entire cartons of ice cream and large pizzas and not feeling full. I became enraged if ice cream was at the wrong temperature and I couldn't eat it fast enough. I snapped plastic spoons with aplomb. One time, I put a pint of rock-solid Ben and Jerry's in the microwave to soften it up. I wasn't sure how long I should set the timer for, and the manufacturer had rudely failed to provide a setting for defrosting ice cream. When the bell rang and I removed the pint, it had melted into ice cream soup. I drank it.

Another time, I bought a box of Snackwell cookies (low fat!), swearing I would not finish them. At most, I'd eat half the box, then save the other half for the next day. I ate three-quarters of the box, barely able to stop myself. I knew the cookies had no chance of making it to the next day, but I was determined not to polish them off. I put the box in the garbage and covered it with trash. Twenty minutes later, I was digging through the garbage, brushing off the box, and devouring the contents.

At a friend's dinner party, I offered to clear the table. When I took the plates into the kitchen, I stuffed the other guests' partially eaten leftovers into my mouth.

One day when I was walking down Bleecker Street, a sexy bakery window caught my eye. I rushed into the bakery, told them I was on my way to a party, and bought two dozen giant cookies. Then I had a private party in my apartment.

Was this behavior normal? I didn't think so. I'd never heard of such things from other people—thin, fat, or anywhere in between.

Listen to Your Hunger

ONE AFTERNOON IN 1994, I found myself in the office of a research scientist on the campus of Columbia University in New York. I was attempting to join an experimental weight-loss study I'd seen advertised in the *Village Voice*. I filled out a questionnaire and then stood patiently while my fat was pinched and measured with calipers by a slightly pudgy scientist in an unflattering white lab coat. I got on the scale. I don't remember what it said, only that it far exceeded my previous top weight of 328 pounds, and that sent me into shock.

The scientist described how the study worked. I'd be given a powder to drink three times a day, and I'd have to return to Columbia weekly to be weighed, measured, and probably pinched by that damn machine again. The powder gimmick was familiar to me, because five years prior, I'd gone on the Medifast protein-powder fast under a doctor's supervision in Rochester, New York, and I'd rapidly shed 110 pounds. I remembered Medifast as my heyday. I wanted to recapture the past glory of losing weight, dropping pant sizes, having friends and coworkers comment on how good I looked. I had obviously forgotten the results of the Medifast program: as soon as I began eating again, I'd regained 125 pounds and wanted to die.

But desperation had led me to Columbia to try another, even stricter, fast. I filled out the medical permission forms with tears in my eyes. If I died, it wouldn't be Columbia's fault, the form said. I wondered if the scientist would come to my funeral, and if he'd be thin enough to button his lab coat when he did.

The scientist told me to report back in three days for a volume-displacement test. As I understood it, he and his grad students would drop me into a tank of water like an overweight ice cube in order to determine my real fat percentage. I imagined my 300-pound body bobbing in a Speedo while skinny graduate students stifled giggles. I set up the appointment, walked out the door, and never went back.

I didn't have another diet left in me. Whatever willpower had previously launched me toward weight-loss schemes had seemingly evaporated. I was empty inside, devoid of any power that might help me control my food intake.

When I walked away from Columbia University that day, I gave up. I couldn't control my eating anymore. I stopped trying to diet, stopped fighting food, and decided to eat whatever I wanted.

At first, the idea was as thrilling as a bungee jump. What would you eat if you could eat anything in the world?

I'd once read a theory about "intuitive eating." It said that the reason people overeat is that they label foods as good or bad, and then they fight to be good. This sets up a pattern of dieting and bingeing that is entirely avoidable. If they simply listen to their hunger and allow themselves to eat without limitations, the theory said, they'd find themselves eating healthy, moderate portions.

Maybe the theory was right, and I'd soon be eating grilled chicken and radicchio salads. Maybe the theory was just an excuse I was using so I could overeat without guilt. There was only one way to find out.

I began to eat without limits, listening carefully to my hunger.

"What do you want for breakfast?" I asked my hunger.

"Two bagels with cream cheese and a Danish," it said.

"Well, all right!" I said.

"What do you feel like for lunch?" I asked it.

"A huge sub, a whole bag of Doritos, and a box of Snackwell cookies," it said without the least hesitation. And, of course, I did what it told me to do.

"Dinner's coming up," I said later. "What are you in the mood for?"

"A dozen hot wings, a chicken burger, and waffle fries with cheese," my hunger said. It also mentioned it had a distinct craving that might be satisfied with a full pint of Ben and Jerry's Chocolate Chip Cookie Dough ice cream.

The "eat whatever I want" plan was fabulous. When I asked my hunger what it wanted, it told me with unerring precision. Unfortunately, what it wanted kept getting bigger and bigger, and my initial joy in eating soon evaporated, replaced with something much more troubling: desperation.

As my food intake increased, my behavior around food got even stranger.

I had never enjoyed buying food in public, but now I tried to avoid leaving the house altogether, ordering in every meal that I possibly could. McDonald's had begun a new delivery service about that time. They had a twenty-dollar minimum. That was fine with me. Three cheeseburgers, a Big Mac, a double cheeseburger, two large fries, two hot apple pies. That was one meal for me.

I had started smoking a few years before, but now I began to smoke like I ate, sucking at the little sticks like a con-demned man, a whole pack at a time. I'd eat until my stomach was near bursting, then I'd smoke until my throat was on fire and I couldn't swallow. Somehow the eating and the smoking were the same thing. They both helped me not think about my life for a few precious minutes at a time.

My promising theater career was in the toilet. Instead of creating plays, I worked as a freelance word processor three days a week, leaving the house only to earn a little money so

I could keep eating. I stopped socializing, preferring instead to spend my time alone with food. I lied to family and friends, telling them that things were going great for me. I learned how to smile when I left the house and how to order small amounts of food on the rare occasion I ate out with other people.

"It's amazing you have a weight problem," they'd say when they saw me dig into a plate of arugula, sun-dried tomatoes, and pine nuts, "because you eat so healthy."

"It's true," I'd say, and I'd smile, already planning the "real" meal I was going to pick up on the way home from the restaurant.

I wore the same pair of pants every day, the only pants that fit me and hid my fat. I never washed them because I couldn't afford to be without them. When they wore out in the crotch, I got a needle and thread and sewed them up. Eventually, my inner thighs were a patchwork quilt of fabric and bad stitching. I walked with my legs squeezed tightly together so nobody would know the truth. I waited at the bottom of subway stairs for the crowd to disperse so I could walk up to the exit without worrying that the person behind me would see marshmallow fat poking through my pant legs.

I began having panic attacks, my heart beating frantically, fear rising like acid in my throat.

It had become an effort to tie my own shoes. It was only a matter of time before I wouldn't be able to tie them at all.

I was no longer a chubby kid, a pudgy teen, or a fat young adult. I was an enormous man. My body ached from the fat. My skin tore, stretch marks crisscrossing my stomach, arms, and chest like ice cracking on a frozen lake.

Listening to my hunger had seemed thrilling at first, but it had devastating consequences for me. Rather than lessening, my eating problem had grown into an immense and terrible force from which it seemed there was no escape.

PART TWO

What I Learned on the Way Down

Sometimes, if you stand on the bottom rail of a bridge and lean over to watch the river slipping slowly away beneath you, you will suddenly know everything there is to be known.

Pooh's Little Instruction Book,
inspired by A. A. Milne

The War Is Over, and I Lost

I SPENT TWENTY-EIGHT years fighting a war against food, fat, and my body. I fought by restricting, dieting, exercising, drinking protein powder, counting calories. I fought by hating myself, swearing I would never overeat again, trying as best I could to keep my promise, then overeating despite myself. I fought battle after battle, and I lost every time. Even when I thought I was winning, I was really losing.

Why couldn't I see the truth?

In hindsight, it's obvious that I didn't know how to stop overeating, but I couldn't admit that to myself. Like a soldier lost in the jungle during battle, I kept fighting long after the war had ended. One day, I finally stumbled out of the jungle, covered in blood, wearing an old army uniform, and people said, "What are you doing? The war ended twenty years ago."

"The war is over?" I said. "I never got the message."

I'm here to give you the message, in case it hasn't been delivered yet.

My war is over. Yours can be, too.

You may not think your war is over. You may think next season's diet will fix you, or an upcoming weight-loss surgery, or a new diet pill. It's possible these things might help you, and I sincerely hope they do. The only thing I know for sure is that they didn't help me. They couldn't help me.

But why?

I'm a Food Junkie

I HAVE A FRIEND who is a recovering alcoholic. She came over to my apartment one afternoon, opened the refrigerator to get a soda, and was startled when a few bottles of beer clinked together in the refrigerator door.

"I didn't know you drank beer," she said.

"I don't really," I said, "but I like to have them around in case friends come over."

The matter was dropped until a month later, when she was over at the house again. She went to the refrigerator to get a soda, and she came back incredulous.

"Those same beers are in there!" she said.

"So what?" I said.

"How long have they been in there?" she demanded to know.

"Maybe nine months."

"Nine months? Are you crazy!?"

We both started to laugh, because we understood how an addict thinks. My friend is hyperaware of beer because it's not

ALLEN ZADOFF

just beer to her. It's a substance that she is addicted to, and it is poison. One sip of beer might set her off on a drinking binge, and the idea that someone could keep two beers in his refrigerator for nine months without drinking them—and without caring—strikes her as absurd.

For a nonalcoholic like me, beer has no power whatsoever. I don't think about it, I don't crave it, I don't remember if there's any in my refrigerator. I'm never sitting at work, watching the clock, waiting for the day to end so I can finally have a beer. On the rare occasion I do drink a beer, I don't want a second beer. I don't even need to finish the first beer.

So it's clear that I'm not an alcoholic.

But let me tell you a story about food.

If You Bite
the Chocolate Bunny,
He May Bite Back

IT WAS APRIL in New York, and I was working at an office in the Flatiron district. I weighed more than 300 pounds at the time. One afternoon our company media director popped into the office where I worked with my five compatriots.

"A client sent me a huge chocolate Easter bunny," she said. "If anyone wants a piece, help yourself. It's on my desk."

My eyes widened.

Free. Chocolate. Rabbit.

I had to have some.

A normal eater who is offered a sugary holiday treat might very well want to try a piece. Indeed, one person in my area got up quickly and walked down the hallway to get some chocolate. Two of the other people said, "No, thanks. I just had lunch."

ALLEN ZADOFF

Me? I started to craft a battle plan.

I waited for the first person to return, then I casually strolled down the hall to eyeball the chocolate rabbit.

The bunny and I saw each other through the office window. She was two pounds, solid chocolate, sitting alone in the middle of the desk and smiling at me. It was love at first sight. I slipped into the empty office, delicately selected a crumb of chocolate that had fallen from the bunny's leg, and placed it on my tongue.

It was delicious. With a twinge of guilt, I casually reached over and snapped off one of her ears. I slid it up my sleeve, and I walked back toward my office.

"How was the chocolate?" my friend Peter asked when I returned.

"It was okay," I said. "Not great."

Without Peter seeing, I slid the chocolate ear out of my sleeve and into my mouth. Almost before I'd stopped chewing, I knew I needed another piece.

I waited as long as I could, and then I stood up. "I think I might get another little piece," I said. "Can I bring some back for anyone else?"

"No, thanks," the assembled coworkers said, and they went back to what they were doing.

I moved down the hall like a lion stalking prey. I slipped into the office and, to my horror, I saw that some other enterprising coworker had already eaten the second rabbit ear. I was outraged, a sense of panic rising in my gut. My rabbit was being consumed by others. Someone was homing in on my territory. If I didn't hurry, she was going to disappear before I could get my share.

I looked for an easy piece to break off the rabbit, but I found I had a big problem. The rabbit was made of solid chocolate, and once her front paws, ears, and bushy tail had been removed, all that remained was a single, thick mass of rabbit body. I scraped at it with my fingernail, but there was no way to get a decent-size piece off of her.

"You just want me for my chocolate," a voice said from behind me.

I whirled around to find the media director staring at me. My face turned bright red.

"It's okay," she said playfully. "I told you to help yourself."

"I'd like to try the bunny," I said, pretending I hadn't already eaten three or four pieces. "But how?"

She looked at the rabbit's body and immediately saw the problem. "Let me grab something," she said.

A moment later, she returned with a butter knife from the kitchen. With some difficulty, she pried off a small piece of chocolate and handed it to me. I popped it in my mouth.

"How is it?" she asked.

"So-so," I lied. "Have you tried it?"

"No. I'm saving room for dinner. Anyway, it's no big deal. I get stuff like this all the time."

It was a big deal for me, not because I hadn't eaten chocolate a million times before, and not because the rabbit was particularly good. It was a big deal because the moment the first piece of chocolate had melted on my tongue, it had set off a reaction inside me that I could not control. I would not be satisfied until two pounds of chocolate rabbit were in my stomach.

I spent the rest of the afternoon peering one-eyed down the hallway, stalking my friend's office, waiting for her to leave her desk. The moment she got up, I was on my feet, speed walking down the hall, maneuvering Wild Kingdom–style past coworkers and bosses, slipping unseen into her office. . . . Time and again I would grip the butter knife in my sweaty fist and attack the rabbit, hacking in a barely controlled frenzy until I released enough chocolate to momentarily fill my mouth. I'd slide out of her office, run a loop around the ninth floor, then circle back to attack again.

I didn't do any work for the rest of the day. Instead, I made half a dozen covert visits to the woman's office, consuming far more than my share of the Easter bunny.

At the end of the day, the media director stopped by our office to say good-bye. Her last words: "I can't believe how popular that rabbit was. It's almost gone!"

Gone but not forgotten.

I can recount a thousand similar stories, some not as obviously pathetic, some a lot worse. I can remember kitchens I lingered in, party tables I stood by, leftovers I flirted with, and drive-throughs I haunted like a hungry ghost. I lied to myself and others about how much and how often I ate. I hid the evidence of my eating as best I could, using thick garden trash bags instead of regular kitchen garbage bags, taking my trash out in the middle of the night, always ordering pizza by the slice in brown paper bags instead of in the telltale pizza boxes that were so difficult to camouflage. I rotated restaurants so countermen would not get to know me and delivery guys wouldn't talk to me.

My behavior was sneaky, secretive, dishonest, and deceptive.

In short, I behaved like a junkie with food.

The Food Fix

IT'S OBVIOUS THAT eating chocolate set up a craving I could not control. But why did I take the first bite of chocolate that day? Was it simply because I liked chocolate?

Of course not. Something else was going on: I hated my job.

I don't mean to say I didn't appreciate the job or realize it was paying my bills. I hated it not because the job was bad but because I wasn't pursuing my dream. My dream was to be a writer, and I wasn't writing. Even worse, I was typing up other people's writing.

You might say I hated myself, hated how I felt inside, and any opportunity to make that pain stop was an opportunity not to be passed up.

I wanted the chocolate bunny that day not simply because I liked chocolate but because I needed it. I was uncomfortable—with myself, with the job, with the day—and the bunny, as crazy as it sounds, looked like the answer to all my problems. I knew that a hit of sugar on my tongue would make my frustration disappear. It wasn't a conscious thought; I knew it in my bones. Eating chocolate meant I wouldn't have to think about the job I resented, the career dream I was ignoring, or the eating problem that was killing me. Enough chocolate, and I wouldn't even remember that I was fat. I would be free.

Such is the power of certain foods, and amounts of food, in my body.

I don't just eat food; I use it. It's my medicine.

It "fixes" me.

But only briefly. Then I have to eat it again. More food, more often.

Unfortunately, I wasn't able to see this while I was overeating. In fact, I wouldn't even begin to understand it until I understood something else first.

I Have a Disease

FOR HUNDREDS OF YEARS, society did not consider alcoholism a disease. People who drank too much were drunks, bums, village idiots. They were the wretched souls who were considered too weak to use moderately a substance that other people easily controlled and enjoyed. Alcoholics lived in darkness, baffled and frustrated, scorned by those who did not understand them. What's worse, they could not understand themselves.

Yet today, when I look up *alcoholism* in my computer dictionary, I find:

alcoholism—an addiction to the consumption of alcoholic liquor or the mental illness and compulsive behavior resulting from alcohol dependency

A Google search hits the following definition:

alcoholism—a primary disorder and chronic disease, progressive and often fatal, where an individual is dependent on alcohol

Two definitions, both right on the mark. It's obvious that the understanding of alcoholism, its causes and effects, has come a long way.

Yet the overeater still lives in the dark ages. Society views the fat person with a mixture of pity and disgust. A little extra weight is allowable, even jolly, but cross the invisible barrier between stocky and fat, and the story quickly changes. A serious overeater becomes the focus of unwanted attention, sidelong glances, advice giving from strangers. Society, frightened by excesses of weight in a body-obsessed culture, looks on the fat person as weak, sloppy, undisciplined.

How could someone eat to the point of destroying his body, his health, his social life? With the hundreds of diets, weight-loss centers, and health clubs available, why are there any fat people left in America?

I try looking up the word *overeater* in that same computer dictionary, but there's no such word.

I look up *food addict.* Nothing.

I do a Google search, and I get a hit:

overeat—to eat to excess, especially when habitual

Is that it? An overeater is simply someone who eats too much?

Not in my experience.

The first time a woman suggested that my overeating might be a disease, I laughed in her face.

It seemed like a cop-out to say I had a disease. I could concede that extreme bulimia and anorexia were diseases (after all, doctors called them "eating disorders"), but I was dubious of even those so-called disorders. Why would a woman starve herself to the point of being skeletal? It made no sense. Couldn't she just choose to eat? Likewise with a bulimic—if she hurt herself by throwing up, it seemed like she should just stop throwing up. I knew that when I got food poisoning and threw up, all I wanted to do was stop.

As for me and my fat, I didn't have an "eating disorder" label to hide behind. I figured that I, more than any of them, should be able to put down the fork.

The problem was I couldn't do it.

Then a remarkable series of events led me to a group of people just like me. For the first time, I was introduced to people who did what I did with food. These were not the people I saw at the commercial-diet weigh-ins or picking up their prepackaged food at the diet center. They weren't the well-meaning doctors and nutritionists who looked at me with a mixture of kindness and pity and gave me the information they thought would help me lose weight. They were not the gym rats, coaches, or trainers who wanted me to eat less and exercise more.

These were people who talked honestly about their own eating, starving, throwing up, and exercising. They talked about their failures at dieting. They talked about hiding food, lying, stealing. Some of them described how they'd thrown food in the garbage, then fished it out. They said they couldn't stop eating certain things until they hit the bottom of the bag or the back of the box. Just like me.

They told me that they had been confused and baffled for years, how the obsession with certain foods, with dieting, with trying to control their bodies, had beaten them down.

I listened carefully to these people, and I found myself immediately identifying with them. To my surprise, I heard the same behaviors described by old black women who never graduated from high school and young white girls who went to private school and college. I heard it from Latino men who were raised to be tough and white men who were raised to be lawyers. Educated and uneducated, young and old, fat and thin, rich and poor. Whatever they had, it didn't seem to matter where they were from, what they looked like, or how much money they were worth. They were all suffering in the same way I had been suffering. The behaviors, though varied, were remarkably similar.

Suddenly, I wasn't alone. My own experience, so strange, private, and shameful, was evidently quite common among a certain group of people.

These people called themselves overeaters, and they said they had a disease.

I had the same symptoms as they.

I, too, was an overeater. I had a disease.

Slow-Motion Avalanche

THE DISEASE OF OVEREATING, I was told, had certain characteristics. For example, it almost always gets worse over time.

I wasn't willing to take that at face value.

Had it been true for me? I looked back at my history.

One thing was immediately obvious: I wasn't born at 360 pounds. I was 210 in elementary school, 272 in high school, 328 before graduate school. My weight had clearly gotten worse over time.

When I examined my life more closely, I realized that weight had been only the most obvious of my troubles. There had been many other aspects of the disease, some subtle, some devastating, almost all of which had gone unnoticed at the time.

My food obsession, for example. I had always enjoyed food as a kid, even loved it. But as the years went by, I went from enjoying food to loving food to needing it. Somewhere along the

way, I crossed an invisible line, and food became more important than the event where it was served. I was no longer looking forward to Thanksgiving with my grandparents; I only
wanted to eat the knishes they served as an appetizer. I no
longer cared about Sunday-night dinner with my family; I only
wanted to sit in front of a tray of corned beef and an entire loaf
of rye bread. And God help my brother if he tried to snag so
much as a potato chip from my plate.

My obsession grew over time, shifting from food to food. I
stalked the local delis in New York, hyperaware of the Entenmann's delivery schedule, knowing the day the Raspberry
Twist Danish would be the freshest. One month I'd be fixated
on donut holes, the next chocolate raisins, the next chicken
wings. My food obsession drifted like a butterfly in the wind,
alighting and clinging to whatever crossed its path.

I began to obsess over the perfect combinations of foods.
Like a mad chemist, I combined sweet and salty and rich and
creamy, layering flavors and sensations in my mouth. Potato
chips were good, but they were better when you mixed them
with pretzels. Bananas were delicious, but when you put them
on a bagel with cream cheese, you created magic.

It's no surprise that many food junkies end up in the restaurant business. We have a natural talent for bringing flavors
and textures together. Unfortunately, I was not able to put my
food creativity to such good use. What began as a playful ex-
ploration with food quickly developed into a personal obses-

sion. It grew to the point that a meal was ruined unless it contained exactly the foods I needed in the amounts and combinations I needed them.

Isolation was another major aspect of my disease. Early on, I realized I was much more comfortable eating alone than I was with people. Still, I enjoyed eating with others, and I could resist the impulse to isolate myself with my food. Over the years, however, I receded more and more from the company of friends and even of strangers. It got so I couldn't enjoy my food if anyone else was around. I simply wasn't able to eat the way I needed to with other people in the room. Eventually, I ate 99 percent of my meals alone in front of the TV. I turned off the phone, locked the door, pulled the shades, and dug into my stash.

My weight obsession also increased over time, the focus on my body growing more acute and judgmental as years passed. My self-obsession developed to the point that I could think only of myself, my needs, and my desires. I had no patience for others or their problems. I detached from the world so I could eat more frequently and without interruption.

When I looked honestly at my past, I could see that in all ways, my disease had gotten worse. What started out as a pebble rolling down a hill had grown to become an avalanche. I'd stood in the center as it came crashing down, not resisting, but helping to pull the earth down on top of me.

The Disease Is
a Triple Threat

AN ADDICT IS someone who reaches for a physical substance to solve a spiritual and emotional problem. There are addicts to drugs, sex, gambling, money, and nearly everything consumable by man.

I am a food addict. That's how I think of myself now and, ironically, it's the key to my eating normally.

If I admit I'm a junkie with food, I don't have to pretend I can eat like a normal eater. I don't have to wonder why I can't have cake on my birthday or candy on Halloween. I don't have to feel bad when I don't join my coworkers for a midafternoon snack or a bite of chocolate bunny.

For years, I didn't understand this. I thought a normal eater's food and my food were the same thing, but they're not. My food is a drug. It's a fix.

And my disease, which I believed to be solely about food and weight, turns out to be much more complex and power-

ful. It's like an Olympic athlete who medals in three different sports in the same Games. My disease has three distinct
and equally powerful components: physical, emotional, and
spiritual.

Fat and Getting Fatter

FIRST, THE OBVIOUS: Overeating is a physical disease. It affects my body.

I overate, and I got fat. I used food as medication, anesthetizing myself with combinations of sugar, salt, and grease. I ate to the point of being sick, experiencing violent cramps, stomach pain, and diarrhea. I used untold amounts of Pepto-Bismol, Immodium, Tums, and Mylanta to try to counter the effects of my eating. I gained and lost weight, indifferent to the fact that such rapid changes in body size and chemistry could have long-term effects on my health.

The disease of overeating is a physical disease, distorting my body, damaging my internal organs, causing me immense physical pain.

The damage is often permanent. It can be fatal.

Because dying from overeating is usually slow and involves many secondary conditions, people misdiagnose it. They call it heart disease, diabetes, or cancer. They shrug their shoulders and say, "He was too young to have a heart attack. What a tragedy."

Nobody says, "He was so fat it killed him."

The physical aspect of the disease also manifests in the fact that I am addicted to certain foods. I call them my "trigger foods" because eating them triggers a dangerous response in my mind and body. One minute I'm nibbling a tiny bit of chocolate, and the next I'm facedown in a chocolate bunny. Thursday morning I taste a sample of something delicious at Starbucks, and Thursday night I have a pastry case installed in my living room.

For reasons beyond my understanding, I cannot eat certain substances like a gentleman. I've never had a handful of Doritos, closed the bag, and called it a day. The only way for me to stop eating Doritos is to cover them with dish detergent and throw them out the window.

It's not just specific foods but overeating itself that is a trigger for me. A normal eater eats too much at a holiday celebration and feels bad. He pushes away from the table, leans back, pats his aching stomach, and says, "I won't do that again for a long time."

For me, overeating has the opposite effect. If I eat too much, I'm compelled to eat more. "I feel like crap," I say. "I'd better have dessert."

My body tells me that the bad feelings associated with being stuffed can be resolved only by eating again until I'm stuffed. It's something like mending a broken arm by breaking the other one.

If you've never been at the mercy of such a process, this will sound absolutely insane to you, and it is. The process is divorced from all logic. When I'm triggered, I am out of control, and I can't think or reason my way out of it. My head says eat. My body says eat. I eat.

In a sense, the early diet-group leaders were correct when they had suggested I identify the burning fuses that led me to overeat. What they didn't know, and therefore couldn't tell me, was that I was suffering from a physical addiction to certain substances and behaviors. As long as I kept practicing these behaviors and putting these foods in my body, the fuses would continue to be lit.

Many diets suggested portion control as an approach to certain foods. Just eat two cookies, they'd tell me, and you'll be fine. But if I could eat only two cookies, I wouldn't have been on a diet in the first place!

The idea of portion control with trigger foods is absurd. It's like doing a little cocaine, three times a day.

This is what I learned about myself. I don't control the triggers; they control me.

Ready, Set, . . . Worry

HOW DO YOU know the difference between a normal eater and an overeater? When a normal eater gets a flat tire, he calls AAA. When an overeater gets a flat, he calls the Suicide Hotline.

This is because the disease is also emotional. As a food junkie, I react to normal life events with a sense of drama and urgency. What would be a minor inconvenience for a normal person is for me an opportunity for Greek tragedy. If you don't return my call, I assume you hate me, and I have to find out why. If you fail to say hello to me in the hall at work, I declare war.

I'm easily hurt. I take things personally. I'm immature. I can nurse a grudge longer than most people own stock.

These are not just my personality quirks. They are the characteristics of many addicts.

While this emotional storm is going on, I'm lost in a narcotic-like haze, eating in a way that makes it impossible to sort truth from fiction. A friend describes the effect of overeating as being covered in bubble wrap. She says the problems of the world hit her softly and then bounce away. Another friend says that when he overeats, it's like he's wearing a diving mask. He's in the world but separate from it, safely ensconced behind a pane of protective glass.

When I'm overeating, it feels as though I'm protected from my emotions, but, really, I'm distorting them. My reactions are inappropriate and out of proportion to the events that caused them. At the same time, I'm numbed out by food, so much so that I'm not able to process my experiences.

The disease of overeating keeps me trapped and immature, relying on food to cope with life.

Entrée Envy

"CAN I HAVE a bite of your pasta?"

At 300 pounds, sitting across from you in a restaurant, I would silently think this question, but pride prevented me from asking it out loud. Instead, I'd eye your marinara like a sad puppy and wait for you to offer me a bite.

Welcome to the third aspect of the disease. I've heard it called "more-ism."

When I'm overeating, I want more of everything: food, love, attention, success, money, sex. Just as appropriate portions of food don't satisfy me, appropriate portions of other human pleasures do not seem enough to fulfill my needs.

Of course, this is an illusion, but it is a powerful one.

One time when I was ten years old, I was eating with my family at the dinner table when my mother said loudly, "Slow down, Allen. Nobody's going to take it away from you." I froze in my seat, suddenly conscious of the way I was eating. I was leaning low over the table, my arms stretched out protectively on both sides of my plate, shoveling food into my mouth at a rapid clip. This was my natural way of eating—quickly and defensively—like a wild animal that fears competition for his food supply.

This was also how I lived my life.

When I was successful, I consolidated the success and guarded it jealously. On the rare occasion I had a girlfriend, I built a perimeter fence around the relationship to prevent my prize from being stolen. When I was young, I secreted away toys so my brother wouldn't play with them. I hid my favorite foods so nobody in the house could eat them.

Protect and defend. It's how I approached nearly every situation.

At the same time I was defending the castle, I lived in constant frustration over not getting enough of what I wanted. In my mind, women didn't love me enough. My peers didn't respect me enough. My creative successes were less than I deserved.

When I couldn't get what I wanted from the world, I took what I wanted from food. A potential employer or mate might tell me no, but a box of cookies never talked back. My eating was a kind of power play, unconsciously designed to seize control from a world that did not play by my rules.

I often had beautiful people and things in my life, but, sadly, I was sick in a way that prevented me from appreciating them. Instead, I looked at what others had, and I envied them. When

I went out to eat with friends and our plates came, I regretted not having chosen their meals. Hence the hungry-puppy act.

We overeaters jokingly refer to this syndrome as "entrée envy." Your food always looks better than mine. But it's not only your chicken parmigiana that looks more delicious—your girlfriend seems prettier, your job better, your success greater. If you have it, I want it. Plain and simple.

Today, I look on this as a form of spiritual crisis—a deep hunger that is seemingly insatiable yet has little to do with food.

"What?" you say. "Eating? Spirituality? Is he crazy?"

Who would imagine that overeating might be a spiritual problem? Certainly not me, and certainly not during the time I was fat. Even now I want to scoff as I write this. Yet my new beliefs grew directly out of my experiences after I stopped overeating. I began to see that what I was trying to fill with food might be better satisfied with other things.

Don't Believe the Hype

FOR OVEREATING TO be recognized as a disease (in my dictionary, anyway), it's going to need some better PR. But in the meantime, it's got a hell of a hype machine at work in my head, and it's churning out press releases night and day. The reason is simple: it wants to eat.

Since it needs me to actually put the food in my mouth, it has to convince me. This is no mean feat when I'm 360 pounds, highly educated, surrounded by doctors and family members begging me to lose weight, and living in a society that often values thinness above all else. To get me to put the fork in my mouth, the disease has an entire publicity department working overtime.

The hype machine will distract me with crazy ideas, filling my head with opinions about myself, my body, and the world. (News flash: You're worthless!)

The machine leads me toward solutions that are not solutions, patiently waiting as I become obsessed with diets.

(News flash: Carbohydrates are evil!) It loves diets, because they keep me focused on food and weight and I never see the big picture. If I don't see the big picture and approach the disease as a physical, emotional, and spiritual malady, I can't fight back.

The machine wants me to become hopeless about my weight. (News flash: Fat people never get thin!) It loves when I read magazine articles about weight-loss trends, and it especially appreciates negative statistics on weight-loss success, including what I see when I get on my own scale. When I look at that number, I become despondent, and the disease's press people can step in and say, "We told you that nothing works. Why are you fighting so hard? Here's a coupon for a free pizza."

The press department for the disease sends me memos telling me there's nobody in the world like me. (News flash: You're alone, and you always will be!) If I start to doubt that it's true, my disease looks around the world and finds evidence— smiling fat people, for instance—to prove it.

If I do meet people who are like me, who understand and share the same symptoms, the disease starts to compare and contrast. It tells me I'm worse than them or not as bad. If you have a disease like mine, for example, then you probably read the chocolate Easter-bunny story and said to yourself, "I've never attacked a chocolate rabbit, so I don't have to read the rest of this book." Or perhaps you saw the list of how much I ate at McDonald's, and you thought, "I've never ordered for three people. I'd better put the book down." (News flash: Allen Zadoff's book doesn't apply to me. Let's go to lunch!)

My disease doesn't want me to read the truth. It will cause me to split hairs when I should be keeping my eye on the big picture. It will have me comparing when I should be identifying.

This is just another trick. The disease is smart, and it wants me to believe the hype, because it wants me on the wrong track for as long as possible. Confusion, diets, quick fixes, self-hatred—they all help the disease accomplish its primary goal: to keep me overeating.

All Eaters Are Not Born Equal

THERE ARE THREE kinds of eaters: normal eaters, problem eaters, and compulsive overeaters.

A normal eater eats when she's hungry and stops when she's full. If she eats a little more over the holidays and gains a couple of pounds, she naturally adjusts after the holidays, and the weight magically disappears. A normal eater is not obsessed with the next meal, the perfect meal, the best dessert in the world. A normal eater is okay with her body. She may not love every inch of it, she may want to make some changes, but she's not stuck inside the house thinking about herself on a summer day. She's at the beach or out with friends having fun.

This is because a normal eater has a normal relationship with food and her body.

A problem eater struggles with food and his weight. He may overindulge on the weekends, then diet on the weekdays. He may be okay for months at a time, then suddenly find he's fifteen pounds overweight and uncomfortable about it. Somewhat grudgingly, he goes on a diet and takes off the weight. Then, buoyed by the compliments of friends, family, and coworkers, he buys new clothes, finds a girlfriend, and leaves the diet behind. He's okay until the next year, when he needs another diet, and the process repeats.

A problem eater thinks about calories. He reads food labels. He tries to make "healthy" choices. He exercises at the gym while doing the math in his head. "One more hour on the treadmill means I can eat a lot at the party Saturday night without feeling guilty," he says. Then he eats too much at the party and feels guilty anyway.

A problem eater may stay a problem eater all his life, or he may get worse over time. He may look back years from now and realize he was already out of control with food but just couldn't admit it at the time. A problem eater may become a compulsive overeater, or he may not.

A compulsive overeater, on the other hand, is obsessed with food and her body, sometimes to the exclusion of all else in her life. She labors under the belief that thin equals well, and she hates herself for not being thin enough. She plans her life around her weight, putting off events until she can fit into a certain dress, swimsuit, or pair of pants. She rewards and punishes herself based on her weight. She doesn't date until the scale tells her it's okay. She eats more when the scale tells her she's got some room to maneuver.

The compulsive overeater often eats to excess and then wonders why she did it. She swears off certain foods and ways of eating only to find herself doing the same thing again the next day. She obsesses over the perfect diet and keeps up on the newest, latest, and best. When she overhears a stranger at work talking about a new and crazy diet, she runs over and has a forty-five-minute conversation with that person. The next day she's on the diet.

A normal eater is free and at relative peace with herself and her body.

A problem eater is struggling, but this struggle has not risen to the level of true misery.

A compulsive overeater has passed through the stages of problem eating to a place of real desperation, unhappiness, and confusion around food and weight. She has lost the ability to control her weight through diet and exercise. Her thinking around food, weight, and body is distorted, and she doesn't even know it.

Normal eater, problem eater, or compulsive overeater: It doesn't matter which one you are. It only matters that you know which one you are.

One Hundred Diets, Zero Success

IF IT'S TRUE that overeating is the symptom of a disease with physical, emotional, and spiritual components, then what's going to happen when I go on a diet?

By controlling my food intake for a while, I suppress the symptoms of my disease. My weight decreases, and I feel better. I'm delighted. I think I'm cured.

What's next? It's time to eat.

This is how it was for me, time and again, diet after diet.

As soon as I went off the diet, the symptoms of my disease came roaring back. Within days or hours, my eating was back up to its previous levels. It didn't matter how much I'd learned during the diet, how much nutrition information I'd been taught, or how carefully the diet tried to ease me down to "maintenance" level. Nor did it matter the promises I'd made, or the joy I felt because of the successful weight loss I'd just attained. When I began to eat again, my eating was quickly out of control. The physical compulsion and mental obsession returned. The weight came back on my body with a vengeance. I was again demoralized, angry, and confused.

In hindsight, I see that dieting was nothing more than a quick fix. Diets were really about one thing: losing weight so I could get off the diet. Nobody goes on a diet with the intention of staying on it for the rest of his life. What I really wanted was to be cured, get off the diet, and go back to—what exactly? I never asked that question. It was too frightening.

The professionals who wanted me to address the *why* of my eating as well as the *how* were on the right track. No diet alone was going to cure me. Unfortunately, those professionals didn't have sufficient understanding of my dilemma, or a process to guide me through the journey. Different people had different parts of the puzzle, but nobody put them together into a cohesive whole. It took other overeaters to do that for me.

When I look back at my dieting history now, I feel sorry for that boy who struggled so earnestly and hated himself for his failures. He was doing his best, but he was lost in the wilderness. He desperately needed a guide.

Today, when I overhear someone proclaiming they have discovered the newest, greatest surefire diet, I can only smile. I know the diet will likely work just fine if the person

is a problem eater but, in the long run, it will be totally ineffective for a compulsive overeater.

If it's true that I have a disease that manifests in emotional,
spiritual, and physical ways, what makes me think I can cure it
by eating cottage cheese for six weeks?

10-90

Diets don't work for me. That was hard news, but eventually I came to accept it. The end of the road occurred when I tried to enroll myself in that final diet study at Columbia University and didn't have the strength to even begin it.

Still, I had a problem with food. A serious problem. So what did I do?

First, I looked at my history and saw clearly that diets and exercise did not work for me. I was trying to change my outsides, while my problem was inside. At the start, this was only an intuition. Later, it was something I began to understand in detail.

Next, I sought help, not with my food intake as I had done so many times before but with the runaway emotions that seemed to be ruling my life and dictating my eating. I knew I couldn't fight alone what had been beating me my whole life. My disease was a combination of Mike Tyson, Muhammad Ali, and George Foreman. I'm just a guy with a decent left jab.

Next, I embraced the idea that I had a disease and that the disease had emotional, spiritual, and physical components.

Finally, I changed my tactics. With the help of others who had done this before me, I focused on my emotional and spiritual development. I put 10 percent of my energy into eating and 90 percent into spiritual and emotional healing.

Think of it: 10 percent into food and eating, 90 percent into healing my life.

No person struggling with an eating disorder would ever believe this could work. After all, the disease manifests in an obsession with food, eating, and body. Obsession is not a 10 percent kind of thing. It's a full-time job, weekends and holidays included.

When I changed my focus, I found my body was restored to normal proportions over time. I didn't lose weight because I tried to lose weight. Weight loss occurred as a by-product of working on other things.

This may sound strange to those not familiar with the process. They will not believe that I could lose weight without trying to control my weight.

I have to admit that I wanted to lose weight. I wanted it desperately. It's not as if I performed some Jedi mind trick and suddenly let go of wanting to be thin. It's just that wanting to be thin and focusing on it had never worked, and I became willing to try it a different way.

At a certain point, I became more interested in eating sanely than in losing weight.

After I lost weight, I did not maintain it by trying to maintain it.

I've done it all very imperfectly. From time to time, I've gotten confused and started to "maintain" my weight. That's what happened five years ago. I thought I was in charge of the process, and I suddenly found myself running around Tokyo trying a bunch of foods I couldn't handle. Twenty-five pounds later, I realized what I was doing and started all over again. ("Are you crazy?" my overeater friend said after he heard what I'd been eating in Japan. "Allen, that was just dessert with an accent!")

When I returned to the United States, I gently shifted my focus back to emotional and spiritual development, and the weight again took care of itself.

Incidentally, I returned to Japan the following year, and I ate sanely and comfortably during a two-month stay in Shibuya, Tokyo. Japan was not the problem, nor was Japanese food. The problem is never outside me; it's always in my head.

10-90 is what's worked for me over the long term. But as I said earlier, there is a strong physical component to the disease, and I cannot neglect talking about the physical aspect of my journey from fat to thin.

That means it's time to move on to the fun stuff.

PART THREE
Food, Glorious Food

"Well," said Pooh, "what I like best—" and then he had to stop and think. Because although Eating Honey was a very good thing to do, there was a moment just before you began to eat it which was better than when you were, but he didn't know what it was called.

The House at Pooh Corner by A. A. Milne

A Note to the Skippers

IF I HAD PICKED UP a book like this twelve years ago, I would have immediately skipped to this part of the book, the section about food. I would probably be reading this chapter while I was standing in the bookstore. I'd be skimming the pages, nervous and spellbound, looking over my shoulder to make sure nobody was watching me. I'd be searching for the recipes, the charts, the secret combination that would unlock the mystery of the Thin Life. When I found it, I'd get so excited I'd run to the coffee shop and have a cappuccino and a chocolate chip muffin to celebrate.

If you're doing that, or if you bought the book and you're reading this part in your living room before having read the rest of the book, let me say a few things:

1. Despite what you think, this is the least important part of the book.

2. If you read the book in order, this part will make a lot more sense.

3. You're not going to find a diet here because this is not a diet book. I'm not going to tell you what to eat. There are professionals who can help you with that.
4. There are no secrets I know about what you should eat. I only know what works for me.

Now, skippers, feel free to read on. Just promise that when you're done, you'll go back and read the book from the beginning.

The Remarkable, Life-Changing, Ultra-Amazing Secret of What I Eat

THERE IS A CHAPTER in every diet book where the author lays out facts and figures, lists "good" and "bad" foods, discloses the secret mix of carbs, protein, and dairy that will get you thin and keep you there for the rest of your life. You're hoping I'll tell you exactly what I eat, and because I lost so much weight, you can eat the same things I did and lose weight, too.

It's not going to happen.

You probably want me to give you a diet. More than a diet. You want a magic formula that will solve your problem forever.

That's not what I have to give.

You want to believe there is a single secret to weight loss, and if you only knew the secret, you'd have it made.

There's no secret.

What I eat is important to me, not at all important to you. My food has varied a lot over the nearly twelve years I've been recovering from the disease of overeating. At times, I've struggled with food, and I've had to adjust what I eat. Something that wasn't a trigger last week or last month suddenly became a trigger, and I had to let it go.

In other words, it's a process, not a solution. Like a boxer, I have to stay on my toes and keep moving, ready and willing to adjust to changing circumstances.

If you took a snapshot of my food every year, you'd have a large and diverse photo album in front of you. That's because my weight loss is based on a variety of factors, all of which are discussed in this book. A food plan is only one small and ever-changing part of that.

My particular food plan is flexible, and it's worked very well for me. But it could kill you.

Instead of telling you what I eat, or thinking I know what you should eat, I'll do something a lot more useful: I'll share some of the things I discovered about food, and show you how I use those discoveries in my life.

Red, Yellow, Green
(and I Don't Mean Salad)

WE'LL START WITH a little exercise.

On a separate piece of paper, make a list of the foods you can't handle. I don't mean the foods you think you should stop eating because they have too many calories. That would be easy: everything you like.

Instead, ask yourself if there are any foods you honestly cannot stop eating once you start. For example, I never ate two bites of a Snickers bar, closed up the wrapper, then forgot about it until the next day. Before I started eating a Snickers, I already knew I was going to eat the whole bar, no questions asked.

So I would put Snickers on my list. Actually, I'd put chocolate in general.

I also have a problem with ice cream. When I was a boy, I'd watch other kids eat ice cream cones, and half of it would end up on their shirts. Yet I could eat an ice cream cone left-handed in a gale-force wind, and I would not lose a drop. Not only did I love ice cream, but I was born with a black-belt skill set in ice cream consumption.

Even today, if you put me in front of a gallon of ice cream with a warm scoop in my hand and asked me to take out an appropriate portion and eat it, I would get the shakes. If you were watching me, of course, I'd take out a single scoop and eat it like a gentleman in front of you. But if you put me in a locked room and gave me a way to hide the evidence . . . different story.

So I would put ice cream on my list, too.

You might be saying to yourself, "I can stop eating any food if I really want to. After all, I'm not eating right now, am I?"

Instead of arguing the point, think about this: What foods do you find difficult to eat in moderation? What foods are no fun to eat in reasonable portions? Can you really eat ten potato chips, walk away, and feel satisfied? If you can, then chips do not belong on your list. But if you close the bag with an internal groan, then secretly look forward to the next time you will open it, put them on the list.

Go now and write these foods down.

We'll call the foods on this list your *Red Foods*.

Now make a list of *behaviors* around the foods that you can't handle. These are the behaviors that cause you to make bad choices, overeat, hate yourself, and so on.

For instance, when I went to a McDonald's drive-through, I used to buy three extra cheeseburgers on top of my regular order. This is because I knew I couldn't be in the car with hot food without reaching into the bag. I ate the cheeseburgers like appetizers while I negotiated traffic on the five-minute drive home. By the time I arrived home, I'd eaten the equivalent of a whole meal in the car. I then ate another whole meal when I got to the safety of my living room.

So I would put eating in the car on my list. Actually, I'd put drive-throughs on the list, too. They were always dangerous for me.

Maybe you're like me, and you too have trouble with eating in the car, or maybe you can't handle salad bars or buffets. Maybe food at parties drives you crazy, or the free samples at the supermarket when you're shopping on Saturday morning.

Perhaps you're undone by tasting while you're cooking, eating while standing up, or eating late at night.

Make your own list of behaviors you can't handle. You might have several, or none at all. If you can't think of any, don't worry. Over the next week or two, they will occur to you, and you can come back to this page and write them down.

Again, make this list quickly, and be as honest as you can.

Let's call these your *Red Behaviors*.

Now make a list of foods that sometimes cause you problems and sometimes don't. For instance, a friend of mine has no problem eating a piece of cake as a dessert when he's at a restaurant with a group of people, but if he buys a cake and brings it into his home, the cake won't make it through the night. He would put cake on his list.

I sometimes struggle with bread. I can have a bagel or roll for my breakfast in the morning, and it doesn't trouble me one bit. But if I start eating sandwiches for lunch, over time I begin to crave bigger and more impressive sandwiches. The desire for bread pushes out my willingness to have a salad or soup or anything else. I don't understand why this is, but it doesn't matter. I put bread on this list.

Maybe you have some foods that you often eat without incident but that sometimes cause you to lose control and abuse the privilege. Maybe you're fine with certain foods when you're happy, but when you're stressed or anxious, these same foods are unmanageable. Write them down now.

Let's call these your *Yellow Foods.*

Now we've come to the last category in the red/yellow/green exercise. This list represents foods that you eat without trouble, guilt, or shame. They are foods you never want to abuse, never cause you problems. They may be foods you consider uninteresting, or you might find them quite delicious. No matter. You're going to put them on the list.

One of my foods in this category is steamed broccoli. I've never woken up in the middle of the night with a craving for steamed broccoli. Hasn't happened yet; probably won't happen in the future. I'm pretty safe with steamed broccoli.

Grilled chicken is another example. I enjoy grilled chicken, but I don't want to eat it until I can't move. One or two grilled chicken breasts is generally enough to satisfy me. This is not the case with fried chicken. One bite of fried chicken, and I'm dressed in a white suit like Colonel Sanders, negotiating the purchase of a chain of KFC restaurants.

I will put *grilled* chicken and broccoli on my list, among other things.

Let's see what's on your list.

These are your *Green Foods.* (The green foods are boring, I know.)

The Traffic Light

You NOW HAVE a list of red, yellow, and green foods and red behaviors.

Think of this list like your own personal food traffic light. Green foods are always go. Yellow foods mean caution. And red foods (and behaviors) stop you dead in your tracks.

Ignore the traffic signals, and you risk accident and injury. Still, if you're anything like me, you want to drive like you're in downtown Bangkok. You speed up when you see a yellow. If there are no cops, you'll run the red light. If it's late at night and nobody's looking, you might just drive up on the sidewalk. What harm could it do?

Plenty of harm, but for now, don't take your lights, or your lists, too seriously. The traffic light is not a secret diet; it's most useful as a tool to help you become aware of what you're already doing with food. You can't change anything if you're not aware of it first.

Pay attention as you eat over the next week, and see if you can identify which foods belong in which category. Come back to the list and add to it. Perhaps you'll find that a food on the yellow list belongs on the red list, or a red-list food is really only yellow. Maybe a green food will be upgraded to yellow. There's no judgment needed here, only an honest accounting of your current relationship with food.

To get an overview, it might help to write the foods on a diagram like the one that appears below.

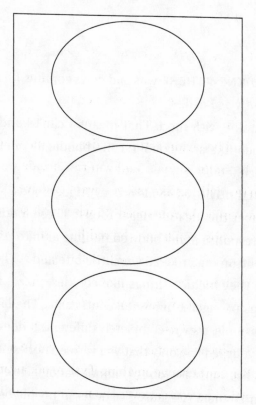

You've done the exercise. You've filled out the traffic light. What now?

Brace for Bad News

YOU KNEW THERE was bad news coming. I'll break it to you as gently as I can.

I'm a junkie with food. That means I can't handle certain foods, much like an alcoholic can't handle alcohol. Can you guess which foods?

That's right. The red foods are my trigger foods.

Remember the idea of trigger foods? These foods trigger a powerful response in my body, something akin to pressing the ignition button on a rocket. One little bite and . . . launch!

For me they include things like cookies, pizza, ice cream, most forms of sugar. Chinese takeout. Pasta. The list goes on. For other people, they're completely different. It doesn't matter what's on your red list, only that you've been honest about it.

My red-list foods are foods I cannot handle. How do I know I can't handle them? Because I've never in my life been able to eat them like a gentleman. With these foods, the serving size listed on the nutrition label is nothing more than a party joke.

I've already told you that my serving of tortilla chips is the bag they come in. I can't eat one cookie; my serving of cookies is the box.

I can't handle these foods because I don't want to eat them in front of another human being. It's no fun for me to eat cookies with you looking at me. I can't eat them the way I want to—by the handful, grunting like an animal.

I am a junkie with food, and the red foods are my trigger foods. That's the way it is. What can I do about it?

Abstain

THIS IS WHAT I do. I abstain from my trigger foods.

abstain—to restrain oneself from doing or enjoying something

I told you it was bad news. I abstain from my trigger foods and also from my trigger behaviors. That means I do not eat the foods or participate in the behaviors.

Your mind is probably in full-scale rebellion. It's saying, "I wrote fried rice down on my red list. I admit I have a little problem with fried rice, but it's not like I'm a junkie with fried rice. I'm not buying it in the park at 3 AM from an Asian chef in a trench coat."

Fair enough. Go and eat some fried rice.

Before you do, call your doctor or nutritionist, and ask her to tell you what defines a reasonable portion of fried rice. Let's say she tells you that a portion is four ounces—the size of a small fist. Go and eat that amount and no more. Eat four ounces. Then stop. See how much fun it is.

When you do this (and I'm quite sure you can do it), you will declare victory over fried rice. Congratulations.

Eat fried rice again, the same portion. In fact, every time you eat fried rice, eat only the exact portion your nutritionist told you. And don't eat it more often than she suggested.

Do this with all your red foods. Ask your doctor or nutritionist what a reasonable portion of each red food is, and ask her how often you should eat it. Then do exactly what she tells you to do.

One scoop of ice cream. Three small cookies. Two slices of pizza. Whatever.

If you can do that forever without anger or bitterness, my hat's off to you. If you can do it without feeling obsessed or wanting more, then I offer you my most sincere congratulations. If you can do it and actually enjoy yourself, not think about it beforehand, not put "Pizza Day!" on your calendar with a green Sharpie, not feel elated in the morning when you wake up and realize it's Waffle Wednesday, then you are free.

You're not a food junkie like me.

If, however, the very thought of eating four ounces of fried rice makes you want to burn down your house, you might be like me.

If the idea of giving up ice cream or some other red food makes you feel like your best friend just moved overseas and you'll be alone forever, you might be like me.

If you think that by eating one brownie and stepping away from the tray you have achieved a miraculous feat on par with the first moon landing, then you might be like me.

If you wonder how you could possibly celebrate your birthday without eating cake, and cake is on your red list, then you might be like me.

An alcoholic will not willingly give up alcohol, and a food junkie like me will not willingly give up his trigger foods. In fact, my mind will do nearly anything not to give up a trigger food. It will lie, justify, rationalize, minimize.

I will write a food down on the red list, then erase it five minutes later because I'm afraid to give it up. Have you erased anything on your red list? Did you avoid putting anything down because you feared I might suggest you stop eating it?

It's okay.

I'm not telling you to stop eating anything. I'm not telling you to abstain from the red foods. I'm telling you what *I* did.

Kicking the Habit

SOMETIMES QUITTING MY trigger foods was like kicking a drug. As I let go of a food, it set off a period of physical and emotional craving, much like that experienced by drug addicts. I didn't need to be tied down or hospitalized, but I did feel like I was going insane, and I needed an enormous amount of support. I dreamed about food, often waking up with a feeling of guilt because I was sure I'd binged. My body ached, and my mind was racked with craving. I felt like I would die if I didn't immediately eat the food in question. I lied and rationalized, trying desperately to come up with any justification that would allow me to eat the food again without guilt.

The good news is that this period of withdrawal was short-lived, and sometimes I didn't have to go through it at all.

Sometimes quitting a trigger food was like blowing on a dandelion. I ate it until I was done with it, and then the need for it just drifted away in the wind.

Whether the process was difficult or easy, once I was off the trigger foods, I was 95 percent free of them. Remarkably, I no longer craved what I had given up. I discovered that eating those foods and trying to manage them was far more difficult than just letting go of them. As my friend Tracie says, "Not an option, not a problem."

From time to time, something would trigger an old desire to eat certain foods. Alcoholics sometimes call these "drink signals." I'd have food signals, briefly feeling the old craving for a particular substance. I found that as long as I had a well-developed system of support in place, and I didn't try to manage these cravings on my own, I didn't have to eat the foods again.

If you are someone who struggles with food, then filling out the traffic light has given you some important information that you may not have known before.

If you feel you are a problem eater (as described in the chapter "All Eaters Are Not Born Equal" in Part Two), you might be able to quit your red foods now that you know what they are. You could even try it as an experiment. "Allen says that when he quit his red foods, he had a little withdrawal, and then he didn't want them anymore." You could try giving up the foods you can't handle, say, for a month. Think of it as wrestling with an alligator. Why do it if you don't have to? You may find that after a period of time has passed, you no longer crave the foods, and you are free.

But if you are a food junkie like me, you will probably be unable to stop eating the red foods and stay stopped on your own. You will keep wrestling the alligator until he tells you he's done with you. I wish it weren't true, but this is my experience. A junkie doesn't wake up one morning, toss his drugs out the window, and spontaneously go clean. I won't say that it's never happened in the history of the world, only that it's a rare occurrence. Every time I quit something in the past, I was back eating it sooner or later.

Ultimately, I did not quit my red foods by deciding to quit them on my own. I did it by focusing on my emotional and spiritual development with the help of understanding people (see the chapter "10-90" in Part Two). That's what led to long-term healing around my food addiction. I'm certain, too, that like an alcoholic, if I put a trigger food in my mouth, I will once again be at its mercy. That's why it's called a trigger food.

Near-Chocolate

We HAVE A delicious sugar-free bakery in Los Angeles that creates marvelous desserts, many of them fruit juice sweetened, dairy free, wheat free. At all times of the day and night, you'll find overeaters, bulimics, and anorexics waiting in line there to purchase their healthy treats. You can easily identify them. They're the ones sweating, staring glassy-eyed at the display case, biting their fingernails.

I call this bakery the Methadone Clinic.

As I said, a food junkie will not willingly give up her trigger foods. She'll naturally try to find a work-around, often in the form of "substitute" foods. Nonfat yogurt instead of ice cream. Bran muffins instead of blueberry muffins. Sugar-free chocolate instead of Toblerone.

I mention this here not because I have anything against healthy, low-fat, or sugar-free foods or baked goods in general, but because playing the substitution game does not work for me. In theory, it makes perfect sense. You know you're triggered by ice cream, so you try eating sugar-free yogurt instead. Then it backfires, and you soon find yourself craving yogurt night and day. You can't understand why, if it's so good for you and it has completely different ingredients, it's driving you crazy.

I can't tell you the scientific reasons it doesn't work. I suspect it's because my trigger foods have a physical *and* psychological component, and I'm just as powerfully addicted to the idea of the food fix as I am to the chemistry in the food fix.

Whatever the reasons, I can't handle wheat-free muffins any better than I can wheat muffins. I'll make myself miserable trying to manage these foods instead of just admitting that they're yet another trigger food that I need to abstain from.

Foods that look like, smell like, and taste like my trigger foods are methadone to me. They're the near-beer (nonalcoholic beer) of the food world.

My alcoholic friends say that if you are an alcoholic and you're drinking near-beer, then you are *Near Beer,* and you should get the hell away from it.

If You Fail to Plan,
You Plan to Fail

LOOKING AGAIN AT my food traffic light, and knowing the red light represents foods and behaviors I can't handle, my path is clear. With the help of a doctor or nutritionist, I create a food plan based on my green and yellow foods.

I secretly know that most of my yellow foods belong on the red list, but I don't worry about that for the time being. I deal with what's killing me the fastest, and I trust that if I stay honest, the details will take care of themselves over time.

Eventually, one of two things will happen: a particular yellow food will turn out to be manageable, or it'll hurt me badly enough that I cry uncle and move it to the red list. Then I'll earn the privilege of abstaining from it, too.

The red/yellow/green exercise was one of the ways I first gained awareness around my food. Years ago, a version of the exercise was suggested to me as a way to inventory my food, and I created the traffic light as a way of thinking about food and developing a sane and abundant food plan. But what I eat is barely the tip of the iceberg. Equally important is how I eat it.

Three a Day

I EAT THREE MEALS a day with nothing in between. This is the *how* of my food plan. It's extremely simple.

Because it's a plan, it's flexible and sane.

Because it's a plan, it's specific and structured.

Each day I set out to work the plan. I eat three meals made up of the foods I know I can handle. I remind myself of the plan by sharing it with another person. I stay honest about the plan by telling someone at the end of the day what I've eaten.

Mostly I just eat three meals and get on with the business of living. After all, it's just food. Once my basic nutritional needs are met, how important is it?

Very important if I'm stuck in the food obsession. But when I do the work I describe here, food gets put in its proper perspective.

Some days, the plan is like a gold-medal gymnastics routine, carried out brilliantly with what seems like little effort. Other days the plan is a train wreck, and at the end of the day I crawl out of the twisted, burning metal, grateful to have survived.

Most days there's nothing quite so dramatic going on.

How is this plan different from a diet?

First, it's based on principles, not on specific foods or combinations I must eat in order to be okay.

Second, it's something I choose to do, because I know what my life is like without it.

Third, there's no quitting this plan. It is a personal bridge to freedom, a way to eat and live sanely each day. There's no contract to cancel or dietitian to rebel against. If I fall off the wagon, I have two choices: lie there and wait to get run over or climb back on another wagon and keep riding.

Finally, it's a personal plan I developed for myself with the help of professionals and other overeaters who understand overeating as a disease and have helped others break their habit before. There's nobody to impress. I'm not judged as good or bad, successful or unsuccessful, based on how well I do it.

This is my plan. Three delicious, abundant meals made up of foods I can handle.

Food Math

WELCOME TO FOOD Math 101. You will not need a calculator for this class because you've done the calculations a million times in your head. Add the calories from breakfast to the calories from lunch to the calories of that cookie you ate three days ago . . .

I'm tired already.

Here's how I used to do food math:

When I was fat, all meals were interrelated in my mind. I ate a small breakfast so I could have a large lunch. I underate lunch so I could overeat dinner. If I overate dinner, I'd skip the next day's breakfast to try to make up for it.

I was "good" during the week so I could be "bad" on the weekend. I ate a healthy dinner Thursday night so I could eat an unhealthy one on Friday. I ate two snacks on Tuesday promising myself I would not eat any on Wednesday.

Every meal was added to and subtracted from the meal before. Each day's food was added to and subtracted from the day, week, and month before.

Each meal was measured on an invisible scale. If it had increased my weight, I hated myself and swore I would never overeat again. If it decreased my weight, I loved myself and celebrated my success, often by eating more at the next meal.

Sound familiar? This process is what I call food math.

Food math is manipulating calories, amounts, and sizes in order to control one's weight. Like a crazed gambler, I ran the numbers over and over in my head, thinking I was going to find a way to beat the system. Food math felt like it was helping me to stay in control, but it was really the opposite. It was an obsession over which I was powerless.

It's Just Lunch

INSTEAD OF FOOD MATH, I just eat lunch. I don't think about breakfast or dinner. I simply eat the meal in front of me. That's the only meal I'm focused on.

I do the same thing three times a day—breakfast at breakfast time, lunch at lunchtime, and dinner at dinnertime.

It sounds like the simplest thing in the world, but for an overeater like me, it's quite difficult.

Now for the trick.

Let's say I go crazy at dinner and eat an entire turkey and enough stuffing to immobilize a grizzly bear. I do not launch into a series of calculations, plans, and promises. I do not pull out a digital scale and get on it naked. I don't go on a diet. Instead, I do something radical and completely counterintuitive.

I let it go.

I know that dinner is over—good or bad, successful or unsuccessful. It's over.

When breakfast time comes, I eat my normal breakfast, completely unrelated to what I had the night before.

Each meal is its own individual performance with a beginning, middle, and end.

And the good news is I only have to eat one meal at a time.

It's Just Wednesday

THE SAME PRINCIPLE applies to each day's food.

What I eat Wednesday has no relation to what I ate Tuesday or what I will eat Thursday. I'm not owed any food from a small meal last week, nor do I have to undereat to compensate for a big meal last night. I'm not saving up for Christmas dinner in six months.

It's just Wednesday, so I eat Wednesday's food.

Simple. But not easy.

But I Want Tortilla Chips

SOMETIMES I WANT tortilla chips. This would be fine if I was a normal eater who could eat ten chips and call it a day. But I know that tortilla chips are for me a full-contact sport. So this is what I do.

When I wake up in the morning, I commit to eating three meals just for today.

I commit to abstaining from my junkie foods just for today.

My disease does not like this idea. Inevitably, it will say, "To hell with your commitments. I want a bag of Doritos right now."

"You can have a bag tomorrow," I tell my disease. "But today, I choose to abstain from Doritos."

"What do you have against Doritos?" my disease argues. "I happen to love Doritos. Millions of people feel the same way."

"I love them, too," I say. "And there's nothing wrong with them. It's just that when I eat them, they interfere with my life. For instance, it's hard to drive with my head at the bottom of a party-size bag of tortilla chips."

"Whatever," my disease says. "I'm eating them tomorrow."

"Yes, you are," I assure my disease.

When tomorrow comes, I again commit to abstaining from my trigger foods and eating three meals. But it's only for twenty-four hours.

Nobody Ever Starved between Lunch and Dinner

FOR AN OVEREATER like me, it often feels like I'm going to die if I don't eat immediately.

It's 3:00 PM. I finished my lunch at 1:00. My dinner is scheduled for 5:30. My disease starts screaming, "Eat! For God's sake, we're going to die if we don't eat!"

"I'm sorry," I say, "but we don't eat again until dinner."

My disease doesn't like that answer, so it gets tricky. "We could wait until dinner," it says. "But what if we have low blood sugar? What if it's a medical condition, like late-onset diabetes? If we don't eat immediately, we're likely to collapse."

"Fine," I say. "We'll go to the doctor on Monday and have a blood test. Meanwhile, we're not eating until dinner."

"Okeydokey," my disease says, "but if we starve to death before Monday, don't blame me."

The disease is very convincing, but I know the truth. I tried listening to my hunger once before, remember? That's what got me to more than 300 pounds.

My Friend the Scale

WHEN I WAS FAT, the day wasn't over until I'd spent some quality time with my friend the scale.

If the number on the scale was too high, I hated myself, panicked, and immediately went on a diet. If the number was low, I rewarded myself by overeating.

If the number was high, I was a bad person and deserved to be punished. If the number was low, I was a wonderful person who deserved love, success, and happiness.

The scale was not really my friend, but I treated it like my personal Svengali, my most trusted adviser. Worst of all, I believed what it said.

Now I know that living with the scale is no way to live.

When I began my journey toward thin, I bid adieu to the scale. I did not weigh myself before or after I lost weight. Actually, I did not weigh myself for seven years. My pant size stayed the same, so I knew I was at the same weight.

Then, when some old ideas returned and I started to struggle with food, it was suggested that I weigh myself once a month as a system of checks and balances. At that point, I needed to weigh myself as a means of fighting denial. For the past five years, I've weighed myself once per month. I get on the scale, but I have no opinion about what I see there. Instead, I share the number with a friend, and then I promptly put it out of my mind until the next month.

The scale is no longer my friend or my enemy. It's just another member of my support team. The number it shows me—once the thing that determined my value in the world—is now just a tool for me to use on my journey.

The Power of "a Little Hungry"

HUNGER IS AN unfamiliar sensation in my body. This is ironic given that I thought I was hungry all the time when I weighed more than 300 pounds. When I spoke to my hunger, it spoke back and told me what to eat. Naturally, I thought this was what other people meant when they said they were hungry.

What I know now is that my head was hungry. My disease was hungry. My body was quite full.

I experienced real hunger only after I'd lost a lot of weight and my eating had stabilized. I was surprised to find that hunger was a physical sensation, something like getting the flu. When I'm hungry, my body feels weak, slow, a little shaky. I may feel dizzy and have trouble concentrating. The feeling goes away almost instantly upon taking a few bites of food.

It's nothing like the hunger I used to feel. That was head hunger. It was a craving that tore through me like wildfire.

Real hunger is satiated with a healthy, moderate amount of food.

Head hunger is insatiable.

Real hunger comes on gradually, disappears after a meal, and does not return for five to seven hours.

Head hunger is a constant drumbeat that only gets louder. Head hunger is obsessive. It drives me toward a specific food or combination of foods. Shortly after eating, head hunger is back again. This is because head hunger is disordered.

Real hunger is part of the natural order.

There's nothing wrong with feeling a little real hunger. It means everything is working just as it was designed to.

It's a Meal, Not a Masterpiece

I'VE DESCRIBED MY food plan as being made up of three sane, abundant meals, but I don't know if that's the right food plan for you. You may be diabetic, you may be training for a marathon (ah, the joys of the carbo-load!), you may be struggling with anorexia. I have no idea how many meals you should eat each day. You can talk to your doctor and nutritionist about that.

Instead, let's focus on the principle, "Meals with life in between."

What are you here for? I don't mean here in the bookstore or in your living room or wherever you're reading this book. I mean here on earth. Why are you on earth? Are you here to move from meal to meal like a ghost, living only for the next meal, hating yourself for the last one? Are you here to think about food 50 percent of the time and your body the other 50 percent?

Or are you here to live?

If you had asked me that question when I was fat, I would not have been able to answer you.

Today I can. Today, I eat three meals a day, and to the best of my ability, I live my life in between. Meals are the refueling stops along the way, not the destinations.

In the past, I was imprisoned by food. I was not living; I was waiting to eat again. Food obsession was like a parasite that burrowed into my body and slowly took over. Early on, it was no more than a nuisance, and I could ignore it. Later, it asserted itself, eventually taking over completely until there was no Allen left, only the desire to eat.

Today I try to put meals in their proper place and remember that I'm here to experience life—to love, grow, and help others. I'm here to write and tell my stories. A meal is no more than a pit stop before I get back to doing those things. Occasionally, a meal is something more, a shared social experience or a means of celebrating an event with others. But this is the exception. Most meals are not all that important.

When a meal becomes more important than the person I'm sitting across from, I'm out of balance. When the meal is more important than the party I'm at or the holiday I'm supposed to be celebrating, I'm out of balance.

When I was overeating, I was happiest when a meal was a masterpiece—designed, perfected, and devoured. It wasn't only fancy food that made me happy. In fact, I could make a masterpiece out of anything. I remember one time in college when I was overcome with a great hunger late at night. A quick scan of the kitchen revealed only a loaf of bread, a stick of butter, and half a jar of jam. Twenty minutes later, I pulled a hot, crusty dessert from the oven. I had invented Poor Man's Danish.

When I stopped overeating, everything changed. I stopped focusing on meals, and I started focusing on life and the people in my life.

Sometimes I forget, and I start to drift back to the old way. My meals get bigger, more interesting, more exciting. My masterpiece mentality returns, and I think my meals should get coverage in the Arts section of the *New York Times*.

Once I recognize what's happening, I stop myself. I remember that it's my life that's supposed to be interesting, not my food. If I want to experience a masterpiece, I can visit a museum. If I'm looking for excitement and fulfillment in food, it's a sign that something's wrong.

Sometimes It's about Learning to Eat the Cookie (a Note to My Anorexic and Bulimic Friends)

I AM NOT ANOREXIC or bulimic, so I don't pretend to speak for you. I do, however, have many friends who are. I've come to believe that anorexia, bulimia, and overeating are different sides of the same coin. The principles in this book will be extremely useful to all people struggling with any compulsion around eating.

But I must warn you. My experience suggests that anorexics and bulimics will love the red/yellow/green exercise for all the wrong reasons. You'll love it because it tweaks your disease.

"Forbidden" foods. "Bad" and "good" food. Restrictions. Rules.

This is the stuff of the "bulimarexic mind." Don't fall for it. Throw out the damn traffic light and find your own way.

There are as many kinds of food plans as there are people eating them with success.

A friend of mine recovered when she stopped eating diet foods. She said she'd been dieting all her life, and it had nearly killed her. So she began to use whole milk in her coffee, butter on both sides of her bread, and sugar in her cereal. In fact, if a food label said "low fat" she wasn't allowed to go near it. She recovered.

Many bulimics I know begin by abstaining from throwing up. I've heard it called "You eat it; you own it." They start with what's killing them the fastest, the vomiting, then slowly develop a food plan that works for them.

I have an anorexic friend who eats three meals a day and three snacks. She abstains from skipping meals or *skimping* on meals. Her food plan includes eating four foods at every meal, and she says the foods must be on the same plate and touching one another. She, too, recovered from near death.

Another friend eats in moderation whenever and whatever she wants to. She had to remove all restrictions from her food plan in order to begin to eat sanely.

None of those plans works for me because I'm a serious overeater, pure and simple. I found that abstaining from trigger foods while eating only three times a day was extremely important for me. But that's my personal story. Yours could well be different.

What I know is that some boundaries needed to be established around my eating because my disease wanted none, all the better to insinuate itself into, and ultimately take over, my life.

These boundaries look different for everyone. For some people, it is about learning how to eat the cookie. For others, it is about learning how not to eat it.

It's only important to know which side of the equation you are on.

Either way, the goal is the same: sane and guilt-free eating.

The Magic Is Not in
the Food Plan

BY THE WAY, recovering from an eating disorder has almost nothing to do with food.

I know what you're saying to yourself: "Is he kidding? After
writing a whole section about food, this guy has the nerve to
tell me it's not about food?"

Well, it is and it isn't.

If eating is killing you, then you need to do something about
your food. But what can you do, really?

If you're like me, you've tried fighting. You've tried all kinds
of fighting. You've looked at this food thing forward, back-
ward, and sideways. Still, you haven't cracked it.

No surprise there. You lost the war, remember? So what
makes you think you have the power to do anything about
your own food?

PART FOUR

What I Know Now

There are people in the world so hungry that
God cannot appear to them except in the form
of bread.

Mohandas K. Gandhi

A Bagel Never Jumped
into My Mouth

ONE DAY IN 1995, I was walking toward a McDonald's on Eighth Street in New York's West Village. My plan had been to buy healthy food at the grocery store and make myself a nice lunch, but the moment I stepped onto the street, like so many times before, my good intentions were tossed out the window for the siren song of fast food. I started to cry as I walked, knowing I was about to do the thing I didn't want to do, the thing that had been hurting me all my life. Now at more than 350 pounds, this thing was getting near killing me.

Suddenly, I stopped in midstride and turned back toward Washington Square Park. I'd never walked away from a binge before, and I had no idea why I was doing it then. Maybe I wasn't really walking away. Maybe I was going to hijack a pretzel cart. I couldn't be sure.

Five minutes later, I found myself sitting on a bench near New York University, and there was not a pretzel in the vicinity.

It was lunchtime on a warm summer day, and the park was filled with people. Businessmen ate sandwiches from brown paper bags. A line of students bought hot dogs and sodas from a food vendor. A young, good-looking couple shared deep kisses on the grass, while a tattooed man with a pit bull watched them out of the corner of his eye. The park seemed a microcosm of the world, and even in my despair I could see the world was filled with love, joy, and human interaction. Food was a part of it, but no more than a small part.

Did I really live in the same world? The world of the park was rich, yet my own was desolate. Food had become my entire life. I felt doomed to be forever separate from those around me—hiding, eating, growing fatter. Other people lived life and celebrated it, but my sole purpose had become the accumulation of pain-filled, highly caloric days.

Sitting and watching the students go by, longing to be a part of life rather than separate from it, I was struck with an intense sense of déjà vu. I had been here before. In fact, I'd spent my life here.

At ten years old, I'd sat on a hill at summer camp, watching other kids play in the lake because I felt fat and was afraid to be seen jiggling in a bathing suit.

At fifteen, I'd sat on the bench at a school dance, watching other people dance because I thought I was too fat to dance.

At twenty, I'd skipped my college graduation because I didn't want to be seen in public at 320 pounds—ironic, given that a graduation gown was about the only thing that would have fit me at the time. I'd stayed home instead, unplugged my phone, and spent the afternoon listening to the sounds of horns honking and music blaring as people drove to postgraduation parties all over the neighborhood.

At twenty-five, I'd walked the streets of New York with food hidden in my backpack, racing back to my apartment so I could again be in my personal Bermuda Triangle.

Now at twenty-eight, I was on a bench in the park, seeing it all again—but for the first time in perspective. Nothing had changed in my life except the locations where I ate. Nothing was going to change.

I looked at my life at that moment, and I saw it was in ruins. I was an emotional basket case, my social life destroyed, my spirit all but crushed. Overeating had stolen my life, but it had happened so gradually, I'd barely noticed.

Suddenly, it all seemed clear. I'd spent my life attacking my weight problem head-on, assaulting it with willpower. I knew I had to try something different, or I would fail again. I stood up from the bench, and I did something I'd never done before: I started to look for help.

But first, I went to McDonald's and ate lunch. Let's face it— twenty-eight years of overeating doesn't evaporate in a second.

I desperately wanted to lose weight, but I knew a diet plan was not the kind of help I needed. After all, I'd sought help from doctors, dietitians, and nutritionists for years, and they hadn't been able to help me get well. Instead of jumping on the next diet, I had to find a way to heal whatever was broken inside me. Not knowing where to begin, I called my first girlfriend, Julia, and, trying to act casual but with a trembling voice, I asked if she would help me find a therapist who specialized in eating disorders. I didn't know what an eating disorder was exactly, but I had a growing suspicion that I had one.

"Of course I'll help you," Julia said, and in that second, it felt like 150 pounds were lifted from my body and my mind.

This was the first step in a long journey that led to my recovery from overeating.

It was only much later that I was able to look back at that moment in the park with a deep sense of awe. How could I, in the midst of a binge, still half-drunk from a breakfast Danish the size of a bedroom pillow, have had such a profound awareness about my life? What force could have overcome, even for the briefest of moments, the habits that had entrenched themselves in my life for twenty-eight years?

If you're thinking I found God, you're wrong. I was far too skeptical for such a belief at the time. First, I found a kind of truth I'd never known before. Food, which had been a very powerful substance in my life, had no real power over me. A bagel never jumped into my mouth. A muffin never tackled me in the grocery store, pried my jaws open, and forced itself down my throat. A pizza never called me in the middle of the night and said, "Get over here. I miss you."

Food had no actual power, but the disease of overeating was very powerful indeed. If I was going to get better, I needed a way to overcome this seemingly gargantuan force.

You might say that desperation made me open-minded in a way I'd never been before. I stopped battling my food problem alone, and I joined forces with others. It was the best decision I ever made.

Over time, I became open-minded about spiritual matters. I started to believe there might be a power greater than the greatest thing in my life, my hunger for food. This power, whatever it was, first led me to the park bench; then to Julia; then to my first therapist, Zimmer; and eventually to people who were like me and knew how to help me recover from a disease I didn't even know was a disease.

A close friend says that the idea of God is too abstract for her, and in order to have a spiritual experience, she needed to find "a God with skin." For her, God only speaks through people. It's by opening herself to the love and ideas of others that she's able to access a power that keeps her from hurting herself with food.

Another overeater friend has her own unique definition of God. She says that God is the three-second pause between the desire to eat and the physical act of putting food in her mouth. That pause did not exist for her when she was overeating, but she has access to it today. In those three seconds, her hand no longer goes immediately to her mouth. That's all the evidence she needs of a higher power.

My own idea of God changes from day to day, varying from the abstract to the human, to the ridiculous, to the divine. I've found it really doesn't matter what I believe. At least, a specific belief is not required in order to recover from the disease of overeating.

Some belief, however, has been necessary for me to eat normally day after day. The disease of overeating was such a powerful force in my life that I simply could not fight it on my own. My utter defeat led me to explore an area where I was previously skeptical—more than skeptical.

When I began to believe there might be a power greater than my need to overeat—whether it was a group of people, a set of ideas, a God, or love—I suddenly found the strength to eat normally. But just for Wednesday.

Spiritual Insulin

PEOPLE WHO FIND out I've lost so much weight are amazed and want to know what diet I'm on. "How did you do it?!" is the first thing they say. When they find out I lost the weight twelve years ago, they assume that whatever diet it was, it's over and done. All the better as far as they're concerned. Any diet that works its magic and goes away is a diet they want to know about immediately. They believe, just like I used to, that being fat is something you deal with for a while and then put behind you, like a bad car crash or a divorce.

If it were only that easy.

Being a food junkie is in some ways like being a diabetic. My disease remains active but manageable as long as I remain in daily treatment. If I take my insulin, I'm okay. If I think I'm suddenly cured, I'm in hot water.

Every day of my life, I take a form of spiritual insulin. Unfortunately, it doesn't come in liquid or pills. It's the by-product of work, a process of healing and growth I practice daily around my overeating disease.

I'm constantly talking about my past, sharing the story of what happened, trying to help others who are dealing with similar problems. I tell a fellow overeater what I eat each day, thereby fighting the powerful tendency to keep secrets and slip into denial around food. I work on my emotional development by going to therapy and practicing honesty with myself and others. I try to grow spiritually by working on my own personal connection to a power greater than myself.

I'm doing all of this imperfectly, sometimes quite poorly. But I'm doing it.

If you had told me twelve years ago the amount of work required for me to be thin, I would have driven right to a donut shop and crawled inside the counter. To hell with being thin.

Of course, that was my reaction to most everything back then.

The fact is that recovery from overeating is the best thing that's ever happened to me. It's fascinating. It's fun. It's a lot of work.

When it all seems too much, I just remember what my options are.

The Secret of the
Caesar Salad

ALTHOUGH IN THIS book I talk openly about my history with food and eating, in my regular life I do not wear my eating disorder on my sleeve. Most people have no idea that I was ever fat, much less that I do all the things I describe here on a daily basis. For many of my friends and acquaintances, this book will be the first time they've heard me talk about food issues, dieting, or weight loss.

When I meet a friend for lunch at a restaurant, for instance, I don't get the jitters and break into a junkie sweat. I don't study the menu for nine hours like a Talmudic scroll. I generally order quickly and ask for something like a chicken Caesar salad. When it comes, I most likely eat it in a reasonable way— napkin on the lap, proper fork, no slobbering noises. In fact, I appear so normal around food, the friend might wonder how it is I could have written a book like this.

What she won't know by looking at me is that I have to do a lot of work to be able to order and eat that salad. She won't know I might have already committed to eating a salad the night before. I may have called someone before going to the restaurant to talk about what I was going to do. I might have written in a journal about our lunch and my expectations for it. I may have meditated in the car before I arrived. I might even silently be saying grace before I take the first bite.

It sounds like a lot of work, doesn't it? Especially when we know that a normal eater shows up at the restaurant, glances at the menu, thinks "What am I in the mood for?" and orders the mozzarella sticks.

I have to do all the work I do because when it comes to food, I'm like a man who has suffered a brain injury and forgotten how to walk. He must relearn basic skills and then apply consciousness and effort to a process that is completely natural for everyone else. It takes work for me to eat like a normal eater, but it's the kind of work most people never see.

A Ph.D. in Overeating

IF THEY GAVE out advanced degrees in overeating, I would have received mine long ago. Unfortunately, I cannot get better based on knowledge about my disease. I do not get better by thinking, studying, and researching the disease. I get better by doing things.

Case in point, I'm writing this book filled with information about being a food junkie. You'd think that because I know so much about it, I'd be immune to its effects. That's far from the truth. When I finish my writing sessions every morning, I want to eat like a hungry bear—pack up my PowerBook, knock a beehive out of a tree, and stick my face in the honey.

My disease evidently doesn't like that I'm telling you the truth. It doesn't like that I'm remembering the truth for myself. It says, "You think you know so much about me? Let's go to McDonald's, and I'll show you how much you know."

Writing this book, I have to be doubly sure to take the actions of a recovering food junkie every day, because my knowledge does not protect me. In fact, it's dangerous to me because it leads me to believe that I've got the situation well under control. The truth is that I never have food under control. Twelve years after sitting on that bench in Washington Square Park, I am still just a food junkie.

Book or no book, thin or not thin, it doesn't matter what I know today. It only matters what I do.

My Body Is None of
My Business

IN THE CLASSIC CARTOON, a beautiful woman walks by a fat man on the beach, and he quickly sucks in his stomach in a vain attempt to win her attention. I was like that guy, sucking in my stomach for three decades, thinking I could win favor and love from the world if only I looked a certain way.

Now, I see that I wanted to control my eating so I could control my body. I thought making my body look a certain way was my job, and I wanted my benefits package to include six-pack abs that would drive the girls crazy. It took me a long time, but I finally accepted that I have no ability to control my body. In fact, during the time I had been in charge of my body, I'd nearly killed myself. I was like a crazed CEO who bankrupts and destroys his company but still won't relinquish power.

Clearly, if I was to get better, I couldn't afford to be in charge anymore.

What followed was a radical shift in perspective. I realized that my body is none of my business, and I started to act accordingly.

What do I mean when I say it's none of my business?

I mean, I don't obsessively monitor my weight. I don't stand in front of the mirror picking at myself, criticizing what I see. If I find myself trying on more than two shirts before leaving the house, I call someone and say, "I'm nervous about where I'm going," rather than wasting time thinking I look too fat to go there.

"None of my business" means I had to give up some old and cherished ideas about what my weight should be. I'd always assumed thin was the only possibility for me, and anything less than thin was unacceptable. In order to get better, I had to allow for the possibility that I didn't know what was best. What if my perfect weight was not 175, but 185 or even 200? What if the perfect weight is what I weigh this very moment?

When I say it's none of my business, I mean that I give up judgments about my body and where it should and should not be. If I feel too fat to go to the beach, I try not to act on the feeling. Instead, I go to the beach and wait for the fat police to throw me out. (Miraculously, it turns out that there is no such thing as the fat police, even in Santa Monica, California!)

Perhaps most important of all, I stop trying to get my body into a certain shape through diet and exercise. I focus instead on my 10-90 strategy, and I let my body transform to the size it's supposed to be, with no extra help from me.

Little Boy, Big Body

USING AN ADDICTIVE substance freezes your emotional development. You think you're growing because the image in the mirror is getting older, but it's an illusion. Alcohol, drugs, food, sex—any substance used addictively—functions like amber, entombing you at the level of emotional maturity you're in when you first begin to rely on the substance.

Overeating seemed like it was helping me to cope with my life, but it was really crippling me. Rather than processing uncomfortable emotions, I was anesthetizing myself with food. I avoided confrontations, choosing to overeat rather than work through conflicts with others. As a result, I never acquired the skills of adulthood.

My body got big, but inside I was a little boy.

Today, I understand that overeating kept me emotionally immature. That's the bad news.

The good news is that when I stopped overeating, I started growing again. Unfortunately, I started where I left off.

One morning after I'd lost a great deal of weight, I stopped at my regular deli on the corner of Sixth Avenue near work. For more than two years, my morning ritual had taken me to this same deli. When I was fat, I had purchased giant pastries and muffins here. Now that I was thin, my order was different, as was my ability to fit through the aisles without turning sideways.

For some reason, there was hardly anyone in line this morning and, before my order was ready, I was standing in front of the young Dominican girl who worked the register. I didn't know her name—we'd never passed so much as a friendly word between us—but I knew she favored gold hoop earrings and tight sweaters, and she never smiled.

"All set?" she said.

"All set."

This was my cue. I would tell her my order, watch her fingers fly across the keys, then avoid her scowl as she snatched my money. But before I could get another word out, she was already ringing me up from memory.

"Do you know what I order?" I said, more than a little surprised.

"It's the same thing all the time, right?"

I nodded, somewhat amazed. I reached for my wallet, and when I glanced up, I found the girl smiling at me.

Was my zipper open? No, the girl was smiling for some other reason I couldn't fathom. Every time I looked at her, her smile seemed to brighten by several degrees. I felt sweat break out on my palms.

"How are you doing this morning?" she said, finally ending the silence.

"Fine."

In two years, she'd never said more than five words to me, but suddenly she was chatting with me like we were old friends.

"You come here every day, don't you?" she said.

"Every day I have work."

I glanced sideways, and I noticed three people waiting in line behind me. I shifted to the left of the register, giving them space to move forward so the girl could take care of them. But when I moved, the girl's head swiveled with me.

"Is there anything else I can get you?" she asked warmly.

"Just a coffee."

"You take sugar?"

"Sweet and Low."

"That's right. You always ask for Sweet and Low. How many do you want?"

"Um . . . three."

Instead of flinging my Sweet and Low into the bag like she usually did, she delicately tore the tops off the pink packages, lifted the cup lid, and tapped them in. This was getting ridiculous. People were waiting impatiently, and this girl was slowly stirring Sweet and Low into my coffee. Had she gone insane?

Finally, my bagel was ready, and she passed it across the counter to me with another killer smile.

"See you around," she said.

"Sure," I said, and I darted out of there with the bag clenched in my hand. I speed walked toward the safety of my office, my face burning, my thoughts racing. Why had the girl been looking at me? Why did it make me feel so uncomfortable when she did it? I was halfway down Twenty-second Street before it hit me: she was flirting with me.

That's why I felt hot, why I was confused, why she had said the same thing over and over again. She was flirting with me, and I'd totally missed it. At twenty-eight years old, I was so inexperienced with women, I didn't even know what it was like to flirt!

I exhibited the same mortifying naïveté in nearly every area of my life. When I stopped overeating, I found I was completely inexperienced at dealing with people and situations in an adult way. Forget adult, I couldn't even deal with them in a teenage way. For years, I'd handled nearly every slight, disappointment, disagreement, and social interaction by walking away and overeating.

Without my junkie foods to rely on, I had a lot of catching up to do.

I Ate Over What
Was Eating Me

You'll REMEMBER THAT when I was fifteen years old, my acting teacher suggested I find out the reasons behind my overeating, and in my quest to become Robert Redford, I tried my best to do what she said.

She thought that knowing why might save me from the misery to come. She was wrong about that, but she was right about something else. Looking at the reasons behind my eating would become an important part of the process of getting to a normal weight. But I couldn't even begin to approach that level of self-analysis while I was still overeating.

When I was acting out as a food junkie, it was impossible to discern my true feelings because I was living a hand-to-mouth existence. Every time I had a feeling, it caused my hand to pick up food and put it into my mouth. This happened so quickly and unconsciously that there wasn't time to ascertain the cause. I didn't know there was rhyme or reason behind my eating because I was too busy chewing.

As soon as I began to eat moderately, the reasons I overate became all too clear. I found that I ate over uncomfortable emotions. In fact, I ate over emotions of all kinds. My eating triggers were hardly limited to bad feelings. Happiness, joy, excitement—stimuli of all kinds—also sent me running for the refrigerator.

What's more, I wasn't just eating over feelings in the moment; I was eating over feelings that were ancient.

Deep, unresolved conflicts lingered from my childhood. Because I'd processed events by eating them out of my consciousness, I had never resolved the majority of my experiences. As my friend says, "When we bury our emotions, we bury them alive." I was stunned to find that all the things I thought I'd avoided—high school shame, sadness over relationships, anger at my parents, jealousy of my younger brother—were waiting patiently for me, sometimes for decades. My mind was like a bus stop in the Twilight Zone. The buses never came, but my feelings lined up for tickets and stayed forever. They smoked cigarettes and ordered from the café, waiting patiently for me to come by and pick them up.

Once I stopped overeating, I had a lifetime of feelings still waiting for their turn to take a ride.

Want to Find Out Why You're Overeating? Stop.

BEFORE YOU RUSH out to your therapist and embark on an amazing journey of emotional discovery inspired by the previous chapter, let me tell you that, in my experience, it probably won't work.

While I'm overeating, I cannot really figure out why I'm overeating. This is because overeating is a narcotic, fuzzing me out and distorting my thinking. While overeating, it is particularly difficult to do the real work of therapy. When I did have therapeutic revelations, they were all but useless to me, especially in the area of moderating my food. Sometimes the revelations were so painful as to lead me right back to overeating again.

I say this even though I am a huge proponent of therapy. Going to therapy has been a critical part of my own process. But overeating is far more powerful than therapy. Doing therapy while overeating is something like trying to ski uphill. You'll put out a lot of effort, but you probably won't get very far.

If you really want to find out why you're overeating, there's one tried-and-true way to do it: stop overeating. And buckle your seat belt, because you just bought a ticket to the thrill ride of a lifetime. Your emotional life is about to become like a ride on Tatsu, the dragon roller-coaster at Six Flags Magic Mountain.

As soon as you stop, you'll begin to experience the feelings that led you to eat. It's built right into the process, or at least it was for me. As my friend Mindy says, "Don't worry about finding your feelings. They'll find you."

Much later, you will consider this an incredible stroke of cosmic good luck. You'll be grateful that it requires no sophisticated techniques to embark on the journey of emotional discovery. You need not meditate ten hours a day, go to a mountaintop, or earn a Ph.D. in philosophy. You need only put down the fork, then get out of the way. And of course, you'll need a lot of help to understand what you find out.

Let me warn you that it won't be pretty. You may feel angry, ashamed, fearful, and sad. You may experience these feelings one at a time, or all at the same time. When I first stopped overeating, my body was racked with sensations I couldn't identify. I ran to Zimmer, my therapist: "Someone criticized me at work yesterday, and suddenly I couldn't breathe, I was pacing back and forth, I wanted to hit him, then I wanted to eat a tray of brownies. What's going on?!"

"It sounds like you were angry," he said.

My mouth dropped open. "Is that what anger feels like?"

Believe it or not, I couldn't identify my own emotions. Overeating was such a powerful narcotic, I'd missed out on the experience of even having emotions.

After a year or so at a normal weight, I began dating Wendy, a social worker who led therapeutic groups for the children of troubled parents. One day she was showing me some of the materials she used with the kids, and I came across a paper filled with cartoon faces, each depicting an emotion—angry, frustrated, bored, excited, and so on. At the bottom of the paper were the words *Today I feel* . . . followed by several empty ovals where the kids could use crayons to draw in their own emotional state. I turned to Wendy and said, "I need a paper like this!"

At twenty-eight years old, I was very much like a child, astonished by every sensation that passed through my brain and body, making the first tentative steps toward self-discovery.

As you might imagine, this felt a lot like going crazy. With my emotions jumping all over the place, I had to wonder why I seemed to be getting worse when I was trying so hard to live a new, healthy life. I didn't yet know that the process of getting sane felt like going insane.

The good news is that the crazy feelings passed with time. My emotions slowed down and lessened in intensity. I was no longer as frightened by my own reactions to the world. Eventually, I could identify feelings while I was having them rather than freezing on the subway platform, on the verge of tears, realizing I was upset by something that was said to me five days before.

Over time, I became adept at identifying and coping with emotions of all sorts. Eventually, having feelings was normal, and my old, sedated way of life seemed a strange and distant dream.

I Eat Because
I'm an Overeater

THE PRECEDING CHAPTERS may lure you into thinking you can "understand" your way to mental health. Before you fall into that trap, let me tell you something else I know now.

Not only do I eat over my feelings, but I also eat for no reason at all.

I eat because I'm an overeater.

The disease of overeating is a shape-shifter, confounding easy explanation. The minute I think I've discovered the secret of why I overeat, I'll find yet another secret. Then another. Then, if I'm really lucky, I'll discover that I'm eating not because of any deep emotional disturbance but because it's Wednesday.

It's folly to think I can figure out the reasons I eat, then head them off at the pass. The journey of emotional discovery is critically important to me as a person, but it's no more than a by-product of my recovery from overeating.

ALLEN ZADOFF

There is a dangerous tendency to mistake understanding the disease with recovering from it. Does understanding diabetes prevent someone from having diabetes?

I'm a food junkie, and a food junkie eats too much. I don't need to know more than that to start getting better.

Life Does Not Begin
at Size 34 Pants

LIFE DOES NOT begin after you can fit into a particular pair of pants. Life does not begin after a diet. In fact, it's happening right now.

For years, I didn't know that. I thought that weight loss would be like the firing of a starter's pistol in the race of life. As soon as I heard the shot, life would commence, and I'd start running. Before that, there was nothing much to do but stretch a little, hang around the locker room, and visualize how exciting the race was going to be once it began. Of course, I had to constantly eat carbohydrates while I waited. I never knew when I might be called on to expend a lot of energy.

There were several problems with this attitude. For one thing, it was no fun. For another, I missed out on nearly everything that was important about the experience of living.

But there was something even more insidious about this belief that I discovered only after I lost a lot of weight.

When 150 pounds had finally melted from my body, my life did not suddenly begin. Quite the contrary. I was confused and upset, afraid of people, unsure of my place in the world. I didn't know how to socialize, have fun, or enjoy myself.

By not practicing living all those years, I had not learned how to live. Now that it was finally "time," I had no skills.

The starter's pistol went off, and I was frozen in place.

I thought I would automatically be happy once I was thin, but that's not what happened. I was thin, but I didn't know how to be happy.

It was time to go out into the world and learn.

Happiness, it turns out, is like a muscle. If I don't exercise it, it atrophies.

Allen Has Left the Building

BEING A FOOD junkie is a little like being a magician. I can make myself disappear anytime. All it takes is a raisin bran muffin the size of a small child. I put it in my mouth, and presto! I'm gone. (If I can't find a muffin that big, I can always press two or three of them together.)

The problem with overeating was not just that it made me fat, but that it changed my behavior. When I ate certain things in certain amounts, I did not want to do much of anything else. My living room became like an opium den in fin de siècle New York. You could find me there twenty-four hours a day, half dressed, slung across the couch, a pretzel rod dangling from my mouth.

When overeating, I became a different person. I limited my social interactions to the minimum possible. I skipped celebrations and parties. I ditched out on appointments. I spent days not answering my phone, not returning calls, not staying in touch with people who needed me. People I needed.

The ironic thing is that all the time I was skipping events, I wanted to be in the world, participating in exciting activities, dating, having fun. It's a particular flavor of hell when you can't answer the phone call of a person who is inviting you to a party because you're busy overeating and dreaming of being at a party.

While I was overeating, I knew I was hurting. I didn't know I was hurting others. People wanted to be my friends, and I wasn't available. They wanted to share their dinner parties, weddings, and celebrations with me, and I didn't go because being in public made me uncomfortable. They wanted to meet me for happy hour, but I was too depressed.

At the time, I thought my pain justified my bad behavior. After all, if you were hurting as much as me, you wouldn't want to make small talk and eat cocktail peanuts either.

I thought I was justified in showing up when and where I wanted, but I was wrong.

When I stopped overeating, I began to clean up the messes I'd made in the past. I couldn't turn back the clock and go to my friend Darrin's wedding, but I could send him a wedding gift and a note of apology three years later. I couldn't return all the calls I'd missed for a decade, but I could do my best to return calls promptly when I received them in the present. (I'm still not great at this. I recently told my friends, I may return only 75 percent of my phone calls, but I answer 100 percent of my e-mail!)

And so, little by little, I have changed my eating and my behavior. When I say I'm going to be somewhere, I am there. It no longer matters if I don't feel like going when the event comes around. I said I'd be there, so I go. End of story.

Eating Well Is My Ticket
to the Show

I EAT THREE MODERATE meals a day not because I want to be thin but because I want to have a life.

Having a normal-size body is nice. Feeling healthier is great. Not hating myself after every meal is wonderful. But all these things are merely side benefits.

I eat sanely so I can live sanely.

I forget this all the time. Maybe a woman I like doesn't like me, or I don't get a job I wanted, and I start to feel ugly inside. Before I know it, I'm feeling ugly on the outside, and I start to think that getting thinner will make me feel better. I decide that I'd like to lose another ten pounds, and I begin to control my food.

This never works for me. The minute I try to eat less, I start eating more. I become frustrated and upset, and the distorted thinking that characterizes my disease kicks in.

It's not until the pain gets bad enough that I remember the truths by which I live today.

I am not a normal eater. My body is none of my business. Spiritual insulin. All that good stuff.

Eventually, my eating returns to normal, and I am again reminded of why I want to eat sanely in the first place. It gives me the gift of being able to participate in my own life. It is my ticket to the show.

A Brownie Saved My Life

I T'S EASY TO think of overeating as a terrible, destructive force. Certainly, it became that in my life, but it didn't start out that way. I'm actually grateful for my overeating, because it got me through some dark days.

When I was unable to deal with the dynamics in my family as a child, food was a safe and readily available means of escape. When I didn't know how to make friends, food was my friend. In adolescence when I was terrified to interact with women, food kept me company.

For a variety of reasons, there was too much trouble and confusion inside me to allow me to easily function in the world. Food kept me safe until I was ready to do the hard work. It was my main coping tool. It was a lover and a friend. It was my therapist, my protector, and my joy. Without overeating, I probably would not have made it into adulthood.

I'm grateful to the brownies for helping me survive. I'm grateful, too, to know that they're no longer the key to my survival.

Warning: Miracle in Progress

I WASTED A LOT of time regretting my past. It was easy to do. I lost a large chunk of my life to the disease of overeating.

I did not have a single date in high school or college. I had sex for the first time at twenty-two years old, followed by many years when I did not so much as touch another human being. I was unable to work at my career. I did not travel. I spent more time in the bathroom than most people spend at their full-time jobs. During my late twenties, I was more or less housebound, living in fear, consuming television and Entenmann's in equal quantities.

My sickness robbed me of so much, and I was angry for a long time. It would have been easy to stay stuck in that anger, but it would have been a tragedy.

When I look at my life today, I see a miracle in progress. If the progress seems a little slow at times, I turn to friends who tell me I'm really growing at the speed of light but I'm just a little too dense to perceive it correctly.

When I look at my past now, I see that for some reason, I was given the awareness of my condition along with the willingness to change. I sought help, and my life, along with my body, was transformed.

I thought you had to be special to have something like that happen to you. I'm just a fat kid from Boston who nearly ate himself to death. Clearly, I did nothing to deserve a miracle, but I got one just the same. Only later did I find out that it's not something you have to earn. It's a gift that is available to anyone who wants it.

Today, I often experience gratitude for the fact that I'm a food junkie. Because of my disease, I've met thousands of amazing people who have survived and thrived with eating disorders. I've found a new way to live in the world with some amount of joy, peace, and fulfillment. I've maintained a normal weight for twelve years. For much of that time, I've been making art, teaching others, and learning about myself. Now I get to tell my story to you.

I've been fat and thin.

I've survived in the dark, and I've lived in the light.

I've had two lives.

How many people can say that?

The Secret of My Success

I SAID EARLIER that an addict is someone who reaches for a physical substance to solve a spiritual and emotional problem. My problem has little to do with food and weight. Those are simply the manifestations of a disease.

My real problem is the way I react to life. I react with fear and trepidation to what most people consider normal human experiences. I deal with that fear by fixing myself with food.

My problem is a living problem. It requires a living solution.

Medication, therapy, exercise, and food plans, all of which are useful tools, do not in themselves represent the solution.

The only solution I have found incorporates emotional, physical, and spiritual healing in equal measure.

The secret of my success is a new way of life.

I wish it were a diet. That would be a lot easier.

This Is Not a
Self-help Book

THIS IS NOT a self-help book because I cannot help my-self. The same brain that had me eating my way to 360 pounds on a sofa in New York will not get me down to a normal weight and keep me there.

They say the definition of insanity is doing the same thing over and over again, expecting different results. I suffer from this particular form of insanity. I believed I could get what I needed from overeating. I kept going back to food long after it had proved itself unworthy of my attention, ineffective as medication, and incapable of solving my life problems.

This is my great dilemma. Overeating doesn't help me live, yet, left on my own, I overeat again and again in a never-ending cycle. This is the essence of being a food junkie.

I cannot break the cycle myself. I must have help.

This book is not that kind of help. It is not meant to be a diet, a system, or a program. I like to think of it as a kind of wake-up call. This particular call might be for you, and it might not. Only you will know.

What I know is that you cannot use what you've read here to stop overeating, undereating, vomiting, overexercising, using laxatives, or any of the myriad forms of eating disorders. I wish I could give you that, but I can't. The best I can do is share my experience and hope that there's something here that might be useful to you.

When I was fat, I, too, read my share of diet books. Each one had me elated, rushing home from the bookstore to scour the pages for a diet secret that might fix me. Each book held the promise of change for my body and my life. Each book seemed like it might be the answer.

If you've read this book, you know that I didn't find my answer in a diet. You may even have some idea why.

My hope is that the ideas contained here may lead you in a direction you haven't tried before. Perhaps these things won't make sense to you now, but they will in a month, six months, or six years. You may well pick up this book again at a later time in your life and find that the lightbulb has gone off. You may even realize the process began when you first read the book.

You may not be able to stop overeating now, but the next time you reach for a food you love and hate, a food you know you shouldn't eat but can't help yourself, perhaps you'll flash back to something you've read here. Instead of hating yourself, you might think, "Maybe it's true. Maybe I have a disease, and the way I'm trying to fight it is not working. Now what am I going to do about it?"

I could not recover from overeating alone. The disease was and continues to be much more powerful than I, and, until I surrendered to it and sought help, I was at its mercy.

Orson Welles is perhaps a strange person to quote here, suffering as he did from his own eating problems, but for various reasons, I think of him now. Bemoaning the incredible difficulty of making films, he once said, "A poet needs a pen, a painter needs a brush, and a director needs an army."

That is my experience with overeating. I need an army to recover from the disease.

Go now and find your army.

Afterword

---

*Though no one can go back and make a
brand new start, anyone can start from now
and make a brand new ending.*

Carl Bard

WHAT YOU CAN DO NOW

I wrote this book to share the story of how I awoke to the reality of my eating and food behaviors. As I said, I had already lost the war with food, but I fought on, oblivious to what had happened. I couldn't see the truth until I was ready to see it.

This book may help you to see your own truth.

After reading it, you may find that you are not like me, and your food and weight problem is still manageable. Perhaps you feel you are a problem eater (see the chapter "All Eaters Are Not Born Equal" in Part Two). In that case, the book may have given you some useful information. For instance, if you know cookies are a trigger food for you, the next time a commercial diet plan promises you can eat cookies for a snack and lose weight, you might politely say, "No, thank you. My own experience with cookies suggests I'd better stay away from them. But I'd like to try the rest of your diet suggestions." You can then embark on the diet with a spirit of gentleness and appreciation for yourself before, during, and after your weight loss.

The book may have also helped you see the ways you've limited your life because of your weight or your perception of it. Perhaps you can start to break down the attitudes that have kept you trapped and hating yourself. The next time you are invited to the beach, you may actually say yes, then show up in your bathing suit with a new thought in mind: "My body is none of my business." You might even enjoy yourself.

Others may recognize themselves in this book and in my experience. We may not be exactly the same in how we deal with food and weight, but my own truths and the thinking processes behind them will be instantly recognizable, and they may make you very uncomfortable. If that is the case, you may suspect that, like me, you are unable to control your own food and weight, and you may even see that all your attempts to do so have ultimately ended in failure.

Perhaps you are an overeater like me. If so, you have an important piece of information that you didn't have before. You may not think so at the moment, but identifying yourself as a food junkie is actually good news. Once you know the real problem, you're already on your way to finding the solution.

If you think you might be a food junkie, or if you already know you are an overeater, bulimic, or anorexic, I suggest you take this knowledge to a medical professional, be it your doctor, therapist, or psychiatrist. Tell them you've read this book, tell them what you found out, and ask for help. If they don't understand (and medical professionals inexperienced with this disorder may not understand), seek another professional, one with more experience in the areas of addiction and eating disorders. Find other food junkies who have recovered and ask them what they did.

The next page lists additional resources that may be useful to you.

Good luck, and remember, you're not alone.

RESOURCES

The following resources offer hope to those struggling with compulsive overeating, bulimia, anorexia, and diet, exercise, and body obsession. The descriptions are from the sites themselves.

Overeaters Anonymous
http://www.oa.org
Overeaters Anonymous (OA) offers a program of recovery from compulsive overeating using the Twelve Steps and Twelve Traditions of OA. Worldwide meetings and other tools provide a fellowship of experience, strength, and hope where members respect one another's anonymity. OA charges no dues or fees; it is self-supporting through member contributions.

National Eating Disorders Association
http://www.nationaleatingdisorders.org
The National Eating Disorders Association is the largest not-for-profit organization in the United States working to prevent

eating disorders and provide treatment referrals to those suffering from anorexia, bulimia, and binge-eating disorder and those concerned with body image and weight issues.

National Institute of Mental Health
http://www.nimh.nih.gov

The National Institute of Mental Health, part of the National Institutes of Health, itself a division of the U.S. Department of Health and Human Services, has a booklet called *Eating Disorders: Facts about Eating Disorders and the Search for Solutions,* which describes in detail the symptoms, causes, and treatments of eating disorders and provides information about getting help and coping.

American Psychiatric Association
http://www.healthyminds.org/

The American Psychiatric Association's *Let's Talk Facts about Eating Disorders* is a brochure designed to reduce stigma associated with mental illness by promoting informed factual discussions of the disorders and their psychiatric treatments.

ACKNOWLEDGMENTS

I'd like to thank the people who made this book possible.

My incredible friends: Tracie Verlinde, Mindy Weiss, Deva Anderson, and Ann Marsh, aka The Posse.

Annalee Autumn Wooster who, in a parking lot one day, said, "Why don't you write a book?"

Stephanie Hubbard, my creative partner in crime, who was present at the birth along with Aomawa Shields.

Julia Martin, my first angel.

My good friend, Peter Mercurio, who may have wanted a bite of that chocolate bunny but didn't get any.

Stephen Zimmer, the amazing Zimmer in the book, who gently and lovingly launched me on my way.

My spiritual brother in NYC, Stephen Adly Guirgis.

Eiko Yamashiro, for her early support of my work at the Tokyo Notice Board.

Ron Burch and David Kidd who have gone above and beyond the call of duty for many years now.

Very special thanks to: Rich Tackenberg, Don Himpel, Roy Levin, Eddie Kehler, Douglas Hill, Daryl Shear, Rebecca Cutter, and Alan Watt.

My agent, Stuart Krichevsky, for taking a chance on an untested writer and working so diligently to bring my story to light. Also Shana Cohen and Elizabeth Coen Kellermeyer at the SK Agency for their help with this book.

I owe a great debt of thanks to Marnie Cochran, who came in at the end of the process and gave the book a home.

Finally, I'd like to thank the many people in New York, Los Angeles, and Tokyo who have taken my calls, listened to my joys and woes, and shared their experience with me over the last twelve years.

This book is for all of us.